V.D. EXPLAINED

No young person should leave school without a sound knowledge not only of sexual relationships, but of sexually transmitted diseases. Two hundred and fifty thousand new patients attend special V.D. clinics each year, and one in every three new cases of gonorrhoea in females is a girl under twenty years old. The author of this book, himself a Consultant Venerologist and clinical teacher, stresses that lack of adequate sex education remains a prime cause of this epidemic. One survey among university girls showed that only 12 per cent had any "reasonble knowledge" of the symptoms of V.D.

This is a practical, honest and workmanlike book, dealing with the origins, nature and symptoms of the various diseases, their treatment and cure. In her Foreword to "Dr. Statham's splendid and informative book" Marjorie Proops says that she receives thousands of letters which "demonstrate the desperate need for knowledge, for practical help and reassurance"—and this need is met with skill and compassion in this important book.

THE CARE AND WELFARE LIBRARY

Consultant Medical Editor: Alexander R. K. Mitchell,
MB, Ch.B, MRCPE, MRCPsych.

V.D. EXPLAINED

ROY STATHAM
MB, Ch.B

Clinical Teacher in Sexually
Transmitted Diseases, University of Nottingham,
and Consultant for Sheffield Regional Hospital Board

with special contributions:

HOW SCHOOLS CAN HELP
Mrs. Kathleen Barratt
A Cambridge headmistress

and

EMOTIONAL FACTORS
Dr. A. R. K. Mitchell
Consultant Psychiatrist

Foreword by

MARJORIE PROOPS, OBE
Daily Mirror

PRIORY PRESS LIMITED

The Care and Welfare Library

The Alcoholic and the Help He Needs   Max Glatt, MD, FRCPsych., MRCP, DPM

Drugs—The Parents' Dilemma   Alexander R. K. Mitchell, MB, ch.B, MRCPE, MRCPsych.

Schizophrenia   Alexander R. K. Mitchell, MB, ch.B, MRCPE, MRCPsych.

Sex and the Love Relationship   Faith Spicer, MB, BS, JP

Caring for the Aged   Dennis Hyams, MB, BS, MRCP

The Autistic Child   I. Kolvin, MD

Aggression in Youth   Roy Ridgway

Stress in Industry   Joseph L. Kearns, MB, B.ch., MSC

Women under Stress   Wendy Greengross, MB, BS, D.obst., RCOG

The Child under Stress   Edna Oakeshott, PH.D

Families under Stress   Brian Phillips, MA, MD

Student Health   Philip Cauthery, MB, ch.B, DPH

The Slow-to-Learn   James Ellis, M.ED.

I.Q.—150   Sydney Bridges, MA, M.ED., PH.D

When Father is Away   The Rev. A. H. Denney, AKC, BA

Health in Middle Age   Michael Green, MA, MB, BCh.

Easier Childbirth   R. E. Robinson, FRCS and B. R. Wilkie, BM, BCh.

Migraine   Edda Hanington, MB, BS

Children in Hospital   Ann Hales-Tooke, MA

SBN 85078 046 2 (Hardback)
    85078 047 0 (Paperback)
Copyright © 1972 by Roy Statham
First published in 1972 by Priory Press Limited
101 Grays Inn Road London WC1
Made and printed in Great Britain by
The Garden City Press Limited
Letchworth, Hertfordshire SG6 1JS

Contents

This book is
dedicated to
Rita

Foreword

by Marjorie Proops, OBE

MANY years ago, when I was at the start of my career as a journalist, I was asked to write a booklet about Venereal Disease for young people. I readily agreed. I needed the money. But while I had a rough notion of what measles and chicken pox was all about, this other disease mystified me.

I telephoned a doctor friend and asked him if he could tell me what kind of a disease this Venereal thing was. He said, very sternly, I thought, "You'd better come and see me right away"—and was enormously relieved to discover why I wanted the information.

It staggers me now to realise that the ignorance about the sexually transmitted diseases among today's teenagers is almost as complete as was mine all those years ago. V.D. may have become a commonplace illness yet it is still surrounded by ignorance and mystique, and by the fear which such ignorance breeds.

As advice columnist of the *Daily Mirror*, I am at the receiving end of thousands of letters which demonstrate the desperate need for knowledge, for practical help and for reassurance.

The kind of questions which come my way illustrate these needs.

"Is it possible to catch V.D. if you let a boy put his tongue inside your mouth when he kisses you?"

"I often masturbate because I haven't got a regular girl-friend. My penis is sore and painful. Do you think I have V.D.?"

"My friend says you can catch V.D. in swimming pools. Is this true?"

A good many adults believe that young people today are very much more knowledgeable than their parents were when they were young. And many young people seem to feel they must put up a great show of sophisticated know-how when they are, in fact, almost as mystified by sex and its various implications as were their parents.

The young cherish the same old myths in which their parents believed.

The big difference between the generations today is that the permissive climate has made it harder for the young to admit their lack of knowledge—and sophistication.

I am convinced that one of the reasons for increasing youthful promiscuity is that all too many of them feel that everyone else is having sex and those who resist it are the odd ones out.

The young may not conform to the standards of their elders—but they conform to the standards set up by their youthful contemporaries. And it's hard not to conform when you are young and insecure.

The gradual decline of close-knit family life, the rejection by so many young people of the values of their elders has increased the need of the young for each other. And what is more consoling than sex? What is more reassuring than sexual intimacy which creates—for the moment at any rate—the illusion of being loved and wanted.

8

"Let me do it," whispers the boy. "I love you. Prove you love me, too." The proof of youthful love can be the subsequent bitter discovery of an unwanted pregnancy, or V.D.—or both.

The diminishing taboos about sex in our present society may have banished a good many inhibitions about sexual intercourse between people of all ages and at all levels of society—but the fearful ignorance about the consequences of promiscuous sex remains.

Sex education, which should be a top priority both in schools and homes, is elementary and frequently non-existent.

The fact that so many young people write to someone like me for help and information is an indictment of our educational system and clear proof of the crying need for the sort of information contained in this book.

The sexual myths must be destroyed. Facts must take the place of fables and old wives' tales. People must understand the risks they take when they join what they think is the trendy "in" crowd. For what they're joining is a sick group—sick both physically and psychologically. And by joining, they spread the message and the sickness.

Sex, says Dr. Statham, in this splendid and informative book, may be a powerful force: it isn't everything, although it seems to be at times.

Certainly when sexual ecstasy is the first step on the road to a V.D. clinic, the ecstasy is soon forgotten in the disappointment of its aftermath.

London,
May 1972

Preface

THIS book is intended to inform young people. It was largely prompted by patients' questions and the often repeated complaint that no one had ever advised them on the subject.

I have attempted to write in simple terms, largely non-medical. Any necessary medical terms are adequately explained in the text. It is hoped that this simple presentation of some of the commoner aspects of sexually transmitted diseases will help young people to make satisfactory decisions concerning sexual practice. If it prevents people from becoming patients then the task has been worthwhile.

I wish to thank most sincerely those who have been kind enough to help in various ways in the production of this work, including:

Mr. J. Coggin and the staff of the Medical Library, University of Nottingham, for assistance in collecting data.

Mr. W. M. Hill, now of the Department of Medical Illustration, Southern General Hospital, Glasgow, and his wife Mrs. R. J. Hill; R. S. Balter, of the Balter Trust; the staff of the Department of Medical Illustration, Nottingham University Hospital Management Committee; Dr. R. S. Morton, Consultant in Sexually Transmitted Diseases for the Sheffield Region and a Disease Control Consultant to the World Health Organisation;

Dr. I. B. Smeddon and Dr. R. E. Church—all these for their help with, and permission to use, illustrations.

Dr. Claude S. Nicol, Consultant in Sexually Transmitted Diseases at St. Thomas's and St. Bartholomew's Hospitals, London, and a Consultant Adviser to the Department of Health and Social Security, for his advice and criticism in the preparation of this book.

Mrs. Noreen Baker and Mrs. Pat Melbourne for secretarial and typing work.

My wife—for her forbearance and assistance at all times; and Dr. Geoffrey Eley, Editorial Director of Priory Press Limited, for his supporting work throughout.

ROY STATHAM

Nottingham,
June 1972

Introduction

THE incidence of some sexually transmitted diseases has reached epidemic levels in certain localities. Gonorrhoea is about as common as measles.

Twenty-five years after the end of the last world war, the incidence of some sexually transmitted diseases is today higher than the peak figures recorded in 1945 and 1946 and others show similar rising trends. The seriousness of this is clear if one recognises that in war time there will be more people with sexually transmitted diseases for, among others, the following reasons: full employment, high wages, vastly more female workers, and young men away from home. Under this aura of disturbed "affluence" an over-riding purpose of destruction of the enemy binds each person to his neighbour. In such alien and emotionally disturbed circumstances, morality shifts, conventional social behaviour tends to decline and sexually transmitted diseases increase.

Today, it can be said that the social revolution in which we find ourselves is comparable to civil war. There is, too, much unrest in other countries, contributing to the multiple forces exerting themselves to change our way of life and our future.

In such conditions it may well be healthy for youth to protest at the uncertainty and injustice of present day living—even if their thinking baffles many middle-aged people. But—and here is the danger—protest may take the form of escapism, experimentation and a negative type of non-conformism resulting in rebels without a cause whose main enthusiasm is discontent for its own sake.

This section of the community is unstable and vulnerable to influences which lower human standards. They represent an adverse social index. They may be uninformed, badly influenced or constitutionally inadequate to cope with living, but they are vulnerable.

The large increase in the number of people affected by the abuse of drugs in the past twenty years illustrates one such adverse social index. Other examples are the rise in alcoholism and the increasing annual figures for suicide and attempted suicide.

The increase in the number of people affected by the sexually transmitted diseases presents a comparable index of social disturbance and it is to this aspect of medico-social welfare that we now give particular regard.

I

How Schools Can Help

An educational contribution by
Mrs. Kathleen Barratt, Headmistress of
Netherall Secondary Modern Girls' School,
Cambridge.

ONCE upon a time it was accepted that parents and teachers knew best. Though whether this premise was truly accepted by anyone other than the parents and teachers—even the Greeks had their troubles—I am not too sure! But in the span of my memory, most youngsters allowed their elders to think along these lines. The difference, of course, some twenty or thirty years ago, was that peer group pressure and general social mores tended to keep most real dangers to the adolescent under control. Now, in many instances, they are exacerbated, by society —by mass media—by group pressure and fashion.

Sadly, teachers and parents are often not so well informed as their teenage sons and daughters—or at least young people honestly believe we are not. I'm regretfully reminded of the old joke about the parent who said to his young son, "My boy, I think we ought to have a talk about sex", and the lad replied, "Yes, Dad, what would you like to know?"

Our young people have a seemingly sophisticated

culture which would appear to put us at a disadvantage. We know that there are drugs—how many parents or teachers have any real knowledge of their popular names, what they look like or their effects? Oh yes, we've all heard of "pot", pills and L.S.D. and heroin—but how much do we *know?* Our young people, even school children, certainly in an urban population will have *seen* more than most of us.

We have heard how the old values regarding sexual matters have changed and indeed, I think if we examined ourselves honestly, most of us will be aware of some shift in our own ideas, but then we become aware that younger and younger girls and boys are being tempted, through curiosity and the example of the slightly older brigade, to try out this experience of sex for themselves. There are even older people, who should know better, who encourage our teenagers to think that unless they have lost their virginity by twenty, there must be something odd about them.

It is a bit like starting to smoke when we were young. It was a sign of being grown up and was delightful because we dare not let our parents know. But now many parents accept that their thirteen- and fourteen-year-old children smoke—some even buy the cigarettes for their sons and daughters. Thirteen or fourteen? I saw a mother the other day with a child of nine or ten, handing a cigarette to him and helping him to light it. It is no longer "a dare" to smoke, so the next thing to try is, perhaps, sex or drugs. Parents today accept that eleven- and twelve-year-old girls have boy-friends and that youngsters of thirteen "go steady". There are even parents accepting formal engagements at thirteen years of age. It is too young. Is it any wonder that progressively each year more girls under sixteen—the youngest, I believe, in

1970 were eleven years old—are having babies or seeking abortions? Or that children, some of whom are only thirteen years, are being seen more often at special clinics?

Unfortunately because sexually transmitted diseases were not so common in parents' youth, not enough importance is placed upon the subject. Many parents have despairingly conceded that their young teenagers will experiment with sex and turn a blind eye so long as a baby does not appear, but disease is hardly considered. Are parents to blame? Are schools?

As a headmistress I would beg parents not to be frightened of standing firmly by their principles, to remember that a child allowed too much of its own way *before* adolescence becomes almost impossible to manage *in* adolescence. But I would also ask for an acceptance of the youngster as a person in its own right and would suggest that the greatest bond comes from communication which starts from an early age and continues into adulthood.

As a headmistress I would ask some of my colleagues in schools and colleges to come out from under the sand. At the present moment many schools feel they are discharging their duties merely by teaching the biological "facts of life". Some schools use religious instruction hopefully to promote sexual and community morality. Please do not imagine that I am denigrating either course of action. There is a need to teach the basic knowledge— but I would suggest that to do this in the secondary sector for the first time is too late and to isolate it to separate subject fields is too narrow.

Of course, it has been said, that ideally it should be the parents who teach the child. Agreed—but so many parents were badly taught themselves that often it is a hard and perhaps embarrassing task for them to offer sound knowledge. I have met quite young fathers who believe it is impossible for a girl to conceive on the first occasion she has intercourse! If only parents would be prepared to be open about the subject, to listen, and to talk, to allow their child to confide, without showing embarrassment: and if only some parents would be prepared to recognise that they have areas of ignorance but yet have sound values to offer. I have seen so many problems caused, or increased, by parents who want to be so "with it" that their children push ever harder to discover just where the boundaries lie. The pity of it is that so many of these parents have said in effect, "We are such good friends. My child tells me everything." Don't you believe it—no child, no person, ever tells "everything". And as I heard a group of fifteen-year-olds agree—"We want our parents to *be* parents—not brothers and sisters."

Life has altered to such a degree over the years since the last war and the problems have increased so rapidly over the last ten to fifteen years, that *nothing short of a complete re-think on what we teach, and how we teach it in this vital aspect of living, will do.* Colleges of Education must include this work in their curriculums and not just from a biological standpoint.

In just the same way that sex is, or should be, a happily integrated part of life, so should the teaching relating to this area be inherent in the philosophy of a school. It should be in proportion, neither swept under the carpet nor made too much of. For pity's sake, do not let us, the adults, get hot under the collar about a subject which the younger generation accept without fuss.

I think that whereas the youngsters have become more open on sex, we, the teachers, are often just as reticent as were the teachers of twenty years ago. We have not accepted the youngsters' knowledge for what it is—and so they feel us to be ignorant, lacking in knowledge of life and unable to teach them anything about the way of life as it is today. When they *think* they know it all they are more at risk than when they *do* know it all! And yet—are they happy?

Far too many adolescents are falling prey to the problems that they are too young to bear and too immature with which to cope, for them to be really happy. It is time we took a hand—but there is a danger—we must not say to them in effect "Don't do this, because I say you shouldn't". If we do, we run the risk of them turning away from our teaching. We must help them to come to their *own* decisions on values. Those judgements must be based on knowledge and we must help them towards a sound conclusion. Self-confidence is to be encouraged so that when taking a thoughtful standpoint they will be less likely swayed by external pressures. Let us not be too delicate, or frightened of facing facts and calling a spade, if need be, a bloody shovel!

This subject must have a background of friendliness, responsibility and loving care. At my own school, thanks to a good and sympathetic staff—a most unprudish group —we deliberately aim at an open, broadminded, quite humorous acceptance of life in all its more human elements. But I hope we are shockable, for without the ability to feel shock, one can become callous.

Our "Learning to Live" programme starts naturally in the first year, with the simple, basic facts of life included in a general hygiene course. This because the entrants come from a wide range of junior schools; in some the BBC and ITV programmes on sex education have been seen, but not in others. We do not set out to impart a *serious* message—it is included as just an everyday part of life—which it is. After this I feel free to talk to any youngster if it appears that I should do so, as do my staff.

Girls mature physically at different rates, as is well known, and a word in the right direction at the right moment can make a good deal of difference—especially if one can go straight to the point. Incidentally, I am of the old school which believes we have a responsibility for our young people outside of school as well as inside the four walls. Fortunately, such are our relationships with the parents that we have worked as parent-teacher teams when needed.

In the second year we do not press the subject—indeed I would hate to feel that there was a pressure felt at any level, but in the third year the biological facts are presented in greater depth, including genetics and so on. Contraception, sexually transmitted disease and abortion are mentioned at this stage but not in great detail.

It is in the fourth year with pupils coming up to fifteen years that we put the whole work into a context of personal relationships (I am thinking that this work may well have to be started in the third year). Other subject areas are called in to aid and abet and we try to get the pupils to see this part of living in a context of leading a satisfactory and responsible life. We teach that the possibilities of greater freedom call for greater personal restraint or else unhappiness might well result—unhappiness not only to themselves, but to their parents and friends.

The subject areas we use are English Literature using books such as *A Kind of Loving, The L-shaped Room, A Taste of Honey, Lord of the Flies, Kes,* etc. as well as selections of poetry and plays. Using pop teenage magazines, romantic ideals are contrasted with realism. Geography highlights pollution and the population explosion and in the "Living" programme, not only do we discuss in small groups, sexual and teenage problems, such as the use and abuse of drugs, difficulties which might arise with friends or married couples coming from different social, ethnic or religious backgrounds, but "experts", all well known to the girls, are brought in to help us.

Expert information is forthcoming on contraceptives— and the problems and responsibilities inherent in their use or lack of use—on sexually transmitted diseases—and abortion.

As visitors are brought into school to help with lessons in other subjects, in all year groups, no stress is felt when an outsider comes in to discuss these problems but because of their expertise—recognised by the pupils and because they do not "preach"—their impact is excellent. Relationships with other people are stressed—and in the linked Home Economics Course the girls and some of the boys from the adjoining school, study types of homes, living with in-laws, older people, looking after young children and problems of the aged or handicapped.

A local vicar, well known in the area, and a marriage guidance counsellor (popular with the youngsters as well as their parents) come in for lessons concerned with marriage, in which the ideal partner, roles in marriage, children in marriage and divorce and the new laws are discussed. Visits are made to an ante-natal clinic and the pupils are taught about the statutory and voluntary services which the city offers. They are given knowledge of where to go to obtain help if they are in need, and they themselves take part in community service.

For this work I have the utmost support from the parents. I call upon parents to help whenever needed, and I believe that parents should be encouraged to come into schools. Let us help our youngsters to become responsible, sensible, unembarrassed, well-informed parents of the next generation. We have a duty as teachers—and to help us carry out this duty we badly needed the kind of information now made available "at schools level" in the following chapters of this book.

2

The Sexual Organs

A young person must, in the end, make up his or her own mind about sexual "freedom" but in order that the decision should be balanced and well informed it is necessary to look more closely at sexual function, sexual practice and related diseases.

To start with there is the basic construction and function of male and female sex organs (genitals). They are set close to some of the organs of excretion or waste-disposal and some of the genital organs also have waste disposal as part of their functions.

Figure 1 shows most of the main features of the male genitals and neighbouring skin areas.

In this drawing the foreskin is pulled back to show the underlying parts. Some male babies have their foreskin removed by (circumcision) a doctor because it is too tight. (Adult males who still have a foreskin should normally keep it in the drawn-down position but can pull it right back for washing.

The scrotum is the bag of skin and muscle below and behind the penis. If the muscle is *relaxed* the scrotum and testicles hang down, the left side often lower than the right. This is often related to a thickened collection of veins passing up in the scrotum above the left testis. There are usually no symptoms associated with this condition and it is nothing to worry about. It is called a varicocele. If the muscle is *tense*, the scrotum is drawn up.

EXTERNAL MALE GENITALS

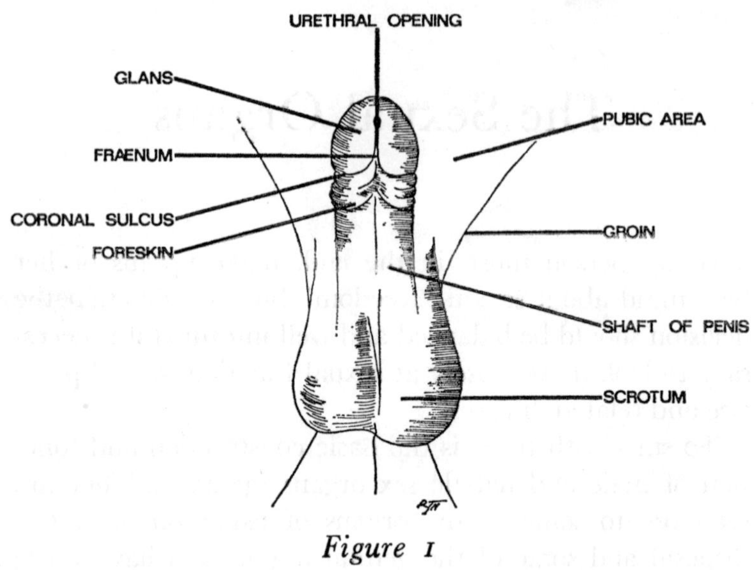

Figure 1

Inside the scrotum are the testicles where sperms (often wrongly called male eggs) are formed.

Figure 2 shows what we would see if we cut vertically straight into the page right down the middle of Fig. 1., and then view the organs from the side.

In Figure 1 the penis was lifted up to show the structures labelled. In Figure 2 the penis is in the normal hanging position and the foreskin is down so that its free border surrounds and more or less covers the urethral opening. The combined function of the male penis and urethra can be seen. The urethra runs down the penis from the bladder and serves as a waste disposal canal for urine. But it is also joined with the sperm tube from the testicle (also known as the testis) and the tube from the seminal vesicle which makes fluid for the sperms to float

SECTION THROUGH MALE PELVIS

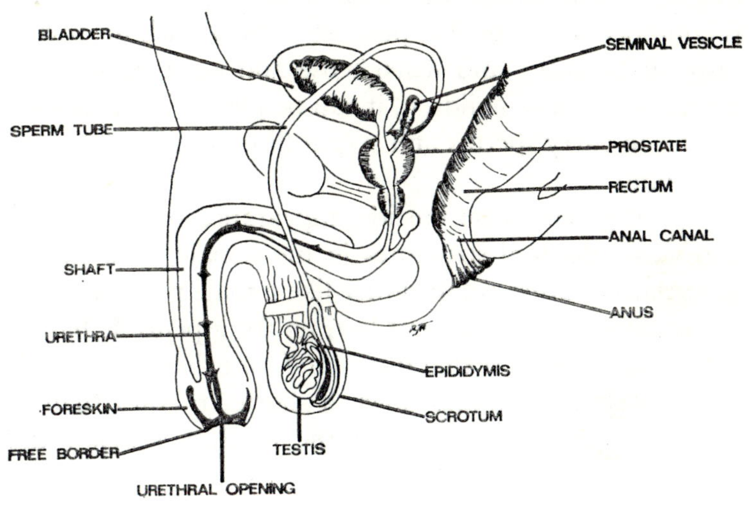

Figure 2

EXTERNAL FEMALE GENITALS

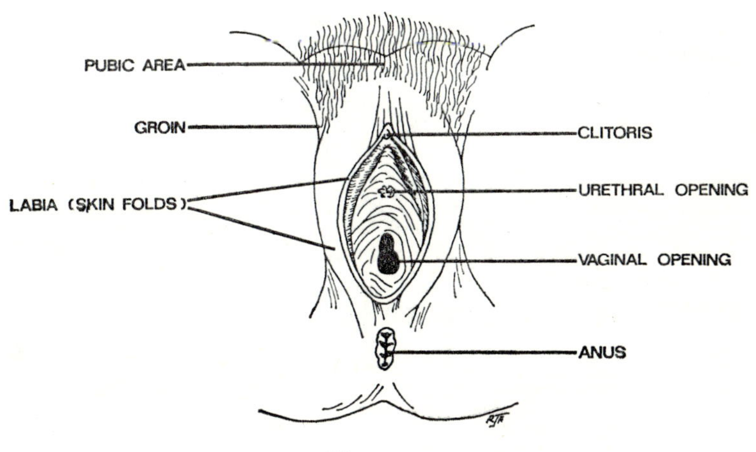

Figure 3

25

in and these are seen connecting with the urethra in the prostate gland under the urine-bladder. Thus the penis is equipped for its double purpose—when slack for waste-disposal of urine, and when tense and erect by nature's design to produce children, it can be placed in the female vagina to carry sperms and sperm fluid to the opening of the womb.

Figure 3 shows the outside appearance of the genital and waste disposal structures in the female. The clitoris is a small sensitive organ rather like a male penis. It plays a part in sexual excitement but, unlike a penis, it has no excretary or direct sexual function. Urine disposal is chan-nelled from the bladder down a shorter urethra than in the male and the opening of the urethra is below the

SECTION THROUGH FEMALE PELVIS

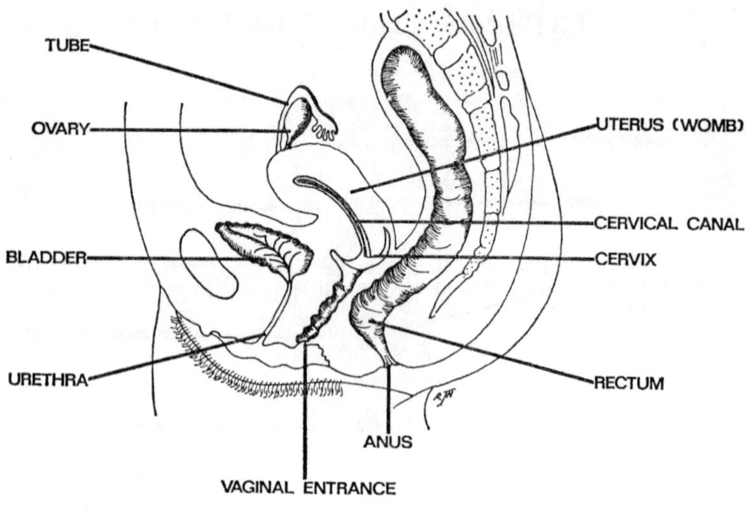

Figure 4

clitoris. Below the urethral opening is the entrance to the vagina, this area and the labia being collectively called the vulva.

As described in Figure 2 for the male organs, Figure 4 shows Figure 3 cut straight down the centre and viewed from the cut side.

At the top of the vagina is the neck of the womb. This is called the cervix and the canal up the middle of it is the entrance of the womb or uterus. The ovary is seen deep in the pelvis. It manufactures eggs which pass down the tube connecting the ovary to the uterus. A sperm deposited in the cervix canal at sexual intercourse may combine with an egg and this starts a baby. The baby grows in the uterus for nine months. At the end of this time the vagina is able to stretch and become wide enough for the baby to pass down and be born.

In Figure 2 and Figure 4 it is seen in both sexes that the back of the pelvis is largely occupied by the rectum where solid waste products collect until they are moved from time to time down the anal canal and out through the exit opening, called the anus.

During the rest of this book the reader may frequently find it helpful to refer back to these drawings and short notes of explanation and function. Also, with this assistance, we can now more easily examine certain sexually transmitted diseases.

Questions and Answers

NOT only people with illness attend clinics. More than one in every five people visiting a special treatment clinic have nothing wrong with them. Many have been at risk. Some have not.

In most respects the fact that such patients attend is encouraging to those who work in this field. Only by patients attending at clinic for specialised tests can early diagnosis be made when disease is present. Correct treatment and cure follow and complications are prevented. This way, spread of disease to other people is also controlled—and in those who are found not to be affected, fears are allayed and much distress prevented.

Venereal Disease (V.D.) is a legal term used by the law-courts and includes only three diseases, namely Syphilis ("pox" in slang terms); Gonorrhoea ("clap") and Chancroid ("soft-sore"). The last named disease is very rare and syphilis is becoming less and less common. At the same time other diseases connected with the sexual organs are becoming much more commonly seen. The term V.D. is thus out-dated and inadequate for the present situation, and as almost all disease of the sexual organs is spread by sexual activity, usually involving sexual intercourse, we use instead the term "sexually transmitted diseases".

Despite considerable publicity recently given to sexually transmitted diseases in the press, on radio and television, many people are still very ill-informed. Furthermore, discussion of genital problems is still difficult for a considerable section of the public. This is due to a variety of factors, perhaps chiefly because of taboos which still exist about genital anatomy and function and because some people feel they cannot find "appropriate words".

Because of these barriers to communication many people delay attendance. This means that those infected have untreated disease for a longer time. The condition may spread further within their body and, of course, they may pass it on to others. In those not affected by disease, delayed attendance at clinic means that unfounded doubts and fears accumulate and increase over weeks, months and even years. Such people eventually do attend a clinic but in varying states of anxiety and real mental suffering all of which could have been prevented by seeking early advice.

It is quite easy to misconstrue variations in normal body appearances. This is understandable. The wide variety of differing marks and structures on the skin of the face and body are well recognised. These areas are commonly or always unclothed and available for inspection and comparison. In our society the genital region is normally covered and genital comparison is not an accepted practice. With the reluctance already mentioned to discuss such features, groundless fears multiply.

Of course, when people by casual sexual contact have placed themselves at risk of disease, then there are real grounds for concern.

Under such circumstances, many find it unacceptable to approach their family doctor. In any case, many family doctors, appreciating the dangers, would refer such patients to a clinic dealing with sexually transmitted diseases. It should also be recognised that the advice of friends may be inaccurate, purposely misleading and frankly dangerous.

Anyone in need of help should attend one of the clinics specially provided for their care. These clinics are widely distributed throughout the British Isles. All cities and reasonably sized towns have them. There are twenty-eight in London alone. By the 1948 Health Act they offer a service wherein specialist advice is available direct to the public. No referral by the family doctor is necessary but the patient may certainly visit their own doctor first if they wish. No appointment is necessary. Clinics are usually held at a variety of times in the week, so that they are equally convenient for shift-workers. The clinic address and times of operation are often advertised in the local public lavatories. If this is not the case, the address and telephone number of the local clinic may be found listed in the telephone directory under "Special Treatment", usually in the hospitals lists.

The unknown is often disconcerting. It will, I hope, be of help before more detailed discussion of individual diseases, if the function and conduct of these special clinics is illustrated by a series of questions often posed by patients, nurses and medical students, followed by the appropriate answers:

1. *Have I got V.D.?* The introduction to this chapter should go a long way towards answering this question. Very often, the patient is really asking in addition:

How ill am I?

Are all the terrible things my work-mates say true?

Is torture part of the treatment: is an "umbrella" really inserted in my penis and then opened?

The best answer to all this is that most of the stories

about sexually transmitted diseases are false. You will be all right if you attend a clinic for advice. And we do *not* use "umbrellas"!

2. *What are sexually transmitted diseases?* These are infectious diseases usually passed from one person to another by close physical contact. Sexual contact or sexual intercourse is almost always involved in their transmission. Those of chief concern are gonorrhoea, non-specific urethritis and syphilis. Different germs which live in, or on, the genital organs or nearby cause different diseases. A small organism called *Trichomonas vaginalis* may cause vaginal inflammation in women or urethritis (inflammation of the urine passage of the penis) in men. A fungus called *Candida albicans* may cause similar diseases.

3. *Can I catch them?* Anyone can catch them by close contact with an infected person. Genital contact or sexual intercourse is usually involved.

4. *How can I avoid them?* By not having sex-contact with a person who is infected. The situation is made difficult by the fact that many women who are infected are unaware of it in the early days and weeks. They have no symptoms or signs and will deny any disease even though they are in fact infected. The same is true in male homosexuals with rectal infection. The use of a condom or sheath on the penis during the whole of the sex act is some protection against becoming infected from an in-fected partner but is not a guaranteed preventive. The problem then remains as to how to be sure that a partner is uninfected.

It should be understood that a person really only knows

one sex life and that is his own. What we know of other people's sex practice depends on what we trust and how much we believe of what we are told.

It follows that infection is least likely where a good and stable relationship exists between only two people as in a satisfactory normal marriage. It also follows that infection is most likely to be transmitted where sex is practised casually and promiscuously.

5. *Which is the serious disease?* This would have applied to syphilis in earlier days, and correctly so. Since modern advances in detection and treatment, serious effects from syphilis are becoming more and more uncommon. The disease may well become a rarity. It is well to remember, however, that if any infection is left undiagnosed and untreated the situation may worsen and greater damage occur. Early diagnosis and treatment are the best methods of control. Diagnosis usually involves special skills and tests using a microscope. The patient should without delay present himself at a clinic organised for such work.

6. *Can I be cured?* The short answer is yes.

For a large number of patients visiting a clinic, diagnosis can be made at their first visit and curative treatment arranged. In some cases diagnosis may involve special additional tests which may take longer but again curative treatment will eventually follow.

Some patients get complications. These are less likely if the patient will attend for advice as soon as he notices any hint of disease.

Non-specific urethritis may recur: probably the patient has to be specially susceptible. In some, a generalised illness can occur although this is not common.

It could be stated here that gonorrhoea cannot recur once treatment has been seen to have cured the infection. If gonorrhoea reappears after cure, then it has been recaught.

7.   *Will it make me sterile or incapable of intercourse?* The short answer is no.

However, if patients do not recognise symptoms and signs of disease or if they ignore them for various reasons, then infection may spread and may lead to genital difficulties later on.

The precaution is early attendance for advice and prompt treatment.

8.   *What do I look for?* The main symptoms and signs of sexually transmitted disease in males are:

(*a*)   URETHRITIS. This is usually denoted by dysuria, an abnormal sensation in the urethra. This varies in different patients from a slight tickling or tingling sensation in the urine passage in the penis, to severe burning pain. This is usually felt most when the patient is passing urine.

The main abnormality which is visible in urethritis is urethral discharge. This may vary from a little opaque off-white fluid to a most marked leakage of yellow or green matter (pus). There may be some blood mixed with the pus. The opening of the urethra may be red and this may extend on to the end of the penis and on to the foreskin in the uncircumcised.

It may be observed here that normal people can feel themselves passing urine. This sensation is increased in certain circumstances, e.g. after holding the urine for a prolonged period so that the bladder is much distended. The normal sensation may also be increased during the

2—VDE * *

first passage of urine after sexual intercourse. The opening of the urethra is normally moist, as are other body cavities. Urine may remain at the urethral opening for long periods after emptying the bladder, especially in the uncircumcised.

Urethritis is concerned with abnormal sensations and discharges.

(*b*) GENITAL SORE. The sore of early syphilis usually occurs on the penis. It may occur nearby or rarely at other areas. As a rule, any genital sore merits special investigation. Obviously a scratch which the patient knows to have been produced by the over-hasty closure of a zip-fastener commands a different approach. A little common sense on the part of the patient should suggest whether attendance at clinic is indicated but if there is any uncertainty, seek advice.

(*c*) RECTAL DISEASE. In male homosexuals, penile symptoms and signs are as above.

Rectal disease may show itself as a discharge and anal irritation. There may be a persistent feeling of wanting to move the bowels, even though this may just have been performed.

A syphilitic sore may be present as a mere crack on the edge of the anus.

If there is any uncertainty, seek advice.

The main symptoms or signs of sexually transmitted disease in females are:

(*a*) NOTHING AT ALL.

(*b*) VAGINAL DISCHARGE. This is a frequent accompaniment of normal life in many women. Some endure considerable degrees of discharge with discomfort and soiling of the clothes without complaint. Any recent change in the discharge may be an important sign of recently acquired infection. Vaginal discomfort of varying degree is sometimes present and this may be marked at intercourse. The surrounding skin may be inflamed.

(*c*) DYSURIA (see definition on previous page) denoting urethritis, as in the male but much less pronounced and less reliable as an indication of disease.

(*d*) As the female often harbours infection for long periods before first being seen at clinic, the infection may well have spread beyond the vagina and urethra. There may therefore also be disturbance of the patient's usual menstrual habit and abdominal pains of recent onset.

(*e*) GENITAL SORE. Any genital sore should receive attention, as described for the male.

Because of the external female genital anatomy, a small sore of early syphilis may pass unnoticed—in skin folds. An internal sore at the top of the vagina is even less likely to be observed unless expert search is made. Even then, it may be overlooked.

9. *How are clinics run?* Patients may attend without referral by the family doctor. No appointment is necessary except in some few clinics where an appointment system has recently been introduced owing to pressure of work. A telephone call to the clinic will ascertain whether an appointment system is in operation. In some clinics patients may be seen privately at certain times. Otherwise the interview with the doctor and the subsequent tests and any treatment necessary are provided under the National Health Service. There are no payments and no prescription charges for treatments given by the clinic.

10.   *What happens when I attend a clinic?* In confidence, personal details are taken and entered in a secret register which is kept under lock and key outside clinic hours. The patient is given a serial number in the register. From then on during his attendances the patient is identified by this number.

This system of calling a patient only by a number was organised many years ago when sexually transmitted disease was regarded as a disgrace and the patients' first thought was secrecy. Names and addresses were never used in public and this is the manner in which most clinics are conducted today. However, social attitudes are changing. Surveys conducted recently in some clinics, notably in London, show that some sections of the public resent being 'numbered' and prefer to be called by their own names. Let it be said that efforts are made to meet patients' preferences.

At interview with the doctor, a history of infection and sexual activity is taken. The doctor is at pains to discover the person who gave the patient the infection so that they too may be traced and treated. Of importance also is the tracing and treatment of anyone whom the patient may have infected since acquiring the disease. Samples are taken from diseased areas and examined in the clinic straight away, thus affording on the spot diagnosis. Specimens are also sent to laboratories for second opinions and special tests. Relevant treatment is prescribed immediately in most cases. Follow-up programme is organised for the patient and for any contacts who are traceable. Blood tests for syphilis are performed as a routine.

Note that a patient should on no account feel embarrassed at the start of the interview with the doctor. Words which are thought suitable may not come readily

36

when required. Patients should realise that they can express whatever they feel wrong in entirely their own choice of words. The doctor will have heard them all before (or most of them!). He may assist the interview with helpful prompting if the patient is hesitant.

11. *How long do I have to attend?* Each patient should attend clinic for a total period of thirteen weeks from the time of infecting intercourse. It should not be assumed that he will have to attend daily or weekly for this length of time. Indeed, he will probably only have to attend about four or five times in all. At the final attendance a last blood test is performed. Only if this test is negative can it be definitely said that the patient is free from syphilis. When the patient attends one week later, providing the blood test is negative, he can be declared free from infection and free from further attendances. This point often proves to be quite a milestone in the patient's life and the great relief produced by discharging the patient from further clinical care underlines the magnified anxieties associated with this field of medicine. It also reminds those working in clinics that patients are at considerable disadvantage. Diplomatic yet dispassionate handling of such a group will achieve best results. Doctors and nurses can do much to allay fears and preserve dignity in the general conduct of clinical management.

12. *Will my family doctor know?* Where the family doctor has referred the patient to clinic with a letter, it is common courtesy and good medical practice to send a reply, saying what has been found and done.

The fact that he was approached first by the patient means that he has been taken into the patient's confidence. It is no disadvantage to the patient if the family doctor receives a report. Indeed, this is probably the ideal situation for he is the medical man in first charge of the patient and it is advisable that he should be aware of his patients' conditions and of any treatment that they are taking.

However, if the patient, for his own reasons, by-passes his doctor and attends clinic confidentially, this privacy is respected and no report is sent to the patient's doctor unless the patient requests it.

13.   *Will my boss/work-mates get to know?* Certainly not, unless the patient for some reason requests it. It should be emphasised that every effort is made to treat patients as individuals and to preserve their due privacy.

On occasion, employers (or school masters) may discover that a person from their establishment is attending clinic. They may telephone the clinic seeking reassurance that the rest of their company are not at risk. In these circumstances due regard to the public health is given and advice may be given over the telephone, at the same time giving little or no detail of the patient's condition.

14.   *Do letters get sent to my home?* No, providing the patient keeps the appointments given to him for his next attendance.

It should be appreciated that a patient with one sex disease is more likely than the rest of the country's population to have contracted another at the same time. Thus, if one disease has been treated and seems to have settled, there is still twofold reason for the patient to continue clinical attendance. Firstly, the treatment, whilst apparently successful at first, may fail after days or weeks and the condition then recurs: this situation requires careful management.

Secondly, while the treated infection may clear up, a second different type of infection may begin to show itself. Patients are only asked to return to clinic a minimal number of times. Clinics are quite busy enough and it can be assured that no-one is asked to attend unnecessarily.

In order to ensure the patients' future health the full survey programme should be completed. If the patient breaks faith and doesn't attend as requested, letters may be sent to his home.

15.   *Can it affect my wife?* An infected man is almost certain to infect his wife at sexual intercourse. A rubber condom or sheath protective gives no guaranteed protection. If intercourse is begun without the use of a sheath, the latter being used only for sexual climax, then it affords no protection at all against sex disease.

When a man has been infected from sexual intercourse outside his marriage he may deny subsequent intercourse for the following reasons:

(*a*)   He doesn't want his wife to know he has had sex with another person.

(*b*)   He may not understand that his wife will have caught the disease.

(*c*)   His wife will probably have no symptoms or signs of disease at all. He reasons that she is therefore perfectly well.

(*d*)   There is a feeling of false hope that, providing he is treated and the infection in him clears up, then the episode can be glossed over and all will be well. But it won't. Eventually, if he has infected his wife, she will begin to show and feel signs of disease and will have to receive attention. And, of course, if *she* is not treated, he will catch the disease back again from her as soon as they resume intercourse!

The situation is more hazardous if the wife is pregnant. During pregnancy wives sometimes do not feel like sexual intercourse with their husbands as often as before. The husband feels rejected and sexually frustrated and may have casual sex outside the marriage. This may be the first time he has done so and on just such an occasion he may well catch a sexually transmitted disease. If he then infects his wife, not only is her health in danger but the unborn baby inside her is also at risk. It thus becomes clear that where a wife has been put at risk by her infected husband, then she must be tested and correct treatment must be provided according to the type of infection found. This is of great importance if she is pregnant as correct treatment will also protect her baby.

Many husbands hesitate to send their wives to a clinic, believing that diagnosis and treatment would best be provided by her family doctor. Some family doctors do go to considerable trouble to make the special tests required for proper diagnosis but they may not have the facilities for doing all the necessary tests. They may also not be equipped to carry through the necessary follow-up programme mentioned previously.

There is also the question of time involved. A family doctor works at considerable pressure to fulfil his commitments in general practice and it is questionable if he should be called upon to undertake specialist responsibilities as well. Special treatment clinics are provided to give this service.

The clinic doctor may interview sexual partners together if they both request it but will not discuss one patient with another without the patient's written permission. Thus, although the domestic management of the situation is the responsibility of the couple concerned, the clinic staff will do all they can to make interviews and treatments as acceptable as possible. It is not the function or practice of clinic doctors and nurses to try to break up partners, whether they are partners in marriage or partners by arrangement.

It may be mentioned at this point, that a pregnant wife may regard herself as, in one sense, protected by her condition and have casual sexual intercourse outside her marriage. Any infection may then pass to her husband. In such cases, if one of a partnership infects the other then they should both attend a clinic where the situation will be handled with understanding.

Changing Pattern

WHILE the number of patients infected with syphylis is gradually becoming smaller, syphylis is a comparatively uncommon disease and its declining incidence does not compensate the growing number of people affected by other sexually transmitted diseases.

The total number of patients attending at special centres in England and Wales is subject to variations over the years. Several influences combine to produce these variations. Thus the return of infected servicemen from abroad at the end of the last world war could be expected to cause a spread of disease and increased numbers of patients attending clinics around the years 1945, 1946 and 1947. In the next few years, a concerted effort to combat these infections with the new drug, Penicillin, again produced a predictable fall in the numbers of patients attending clinics.

A much clearer idea of what is happening to sexually transmitted diseases and sex-habits will be obtained if we set the trends down in small lists of figures.

Some explanatory notes will help easy understanding.

(*a*)   The tables represent the numbers of patients reported in England and Wales in alternate years over the past twenty years. Scotland produces separate figures.

(*b*)   The last available totals at the present time are for 1970. Nevertheless, the trends are obviously upwards and there is no evidence of any alteration in these trends as judged on present clinic attendances.

(c)   The years are divided into two columns. Reading down the left hand set, then the right hand set, gives a quick appreciation of the trend of disease.

(d)   Graphs can be constructed from the tables to give a picture of disease. Graphs are not difficult to understand. Let us say that in one year, say 1968, a disease occurred x times. In 1969 it occurred twice as often, so the figure is 2x. And in 1970, three times as often—that is 3x. Our disease table of figures thus is:

YEAR	PATIENTS
1968	x
1969	2x
1970	3x

A graph of this situation could be drawn as follows and the rise of the graph from left to right shows the upward trend of the disease.

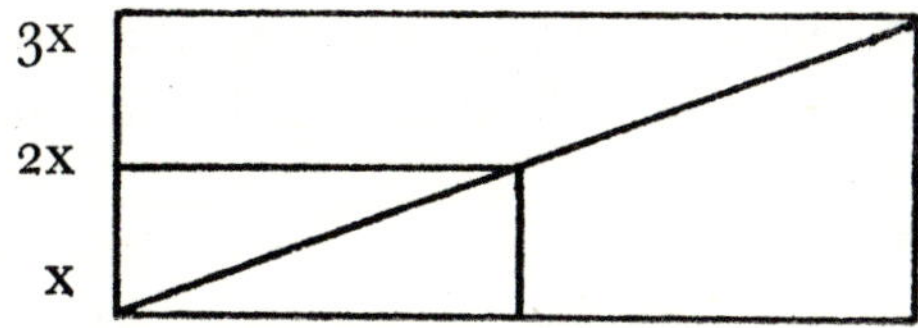

TABLE I

<u>GONORRHOEA</u>

1952	19,095	1962	35,438
1954	17,536	1964	37,665
1956	20,388	1966	37,483
1958	27,887	1968	44,962
1960	33,770	1970	54,764

We can easily appreciate the changing pattern in the incidence of gonorrhoea from Table I. Graph I gives a fuller picture. The high peak at A illustrates how common this disease was at the end of the last world war, as we have mentioned earlier.

The great reduction in cases due to penicillin treatment and other factors is well illustrated down to the comparatively low levels at B in the early 1950s. Point c shows that by 1970 the post-war peak of disease had been passed and the number of patients affected by this disease is still increasing.

The very steep rise in the last three years cannot pass unnoticed. There can be no surprise that in some areas this disease can be called an epidemic and is out of control.

Table II and Graph II indicate similar tendencies in non-gonococcal urethritis in the male. The steep rise in the final year is obvious.

GRAPH I

RISING INCIDENCE OF GONORRHOEA

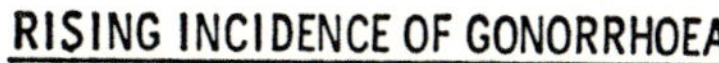

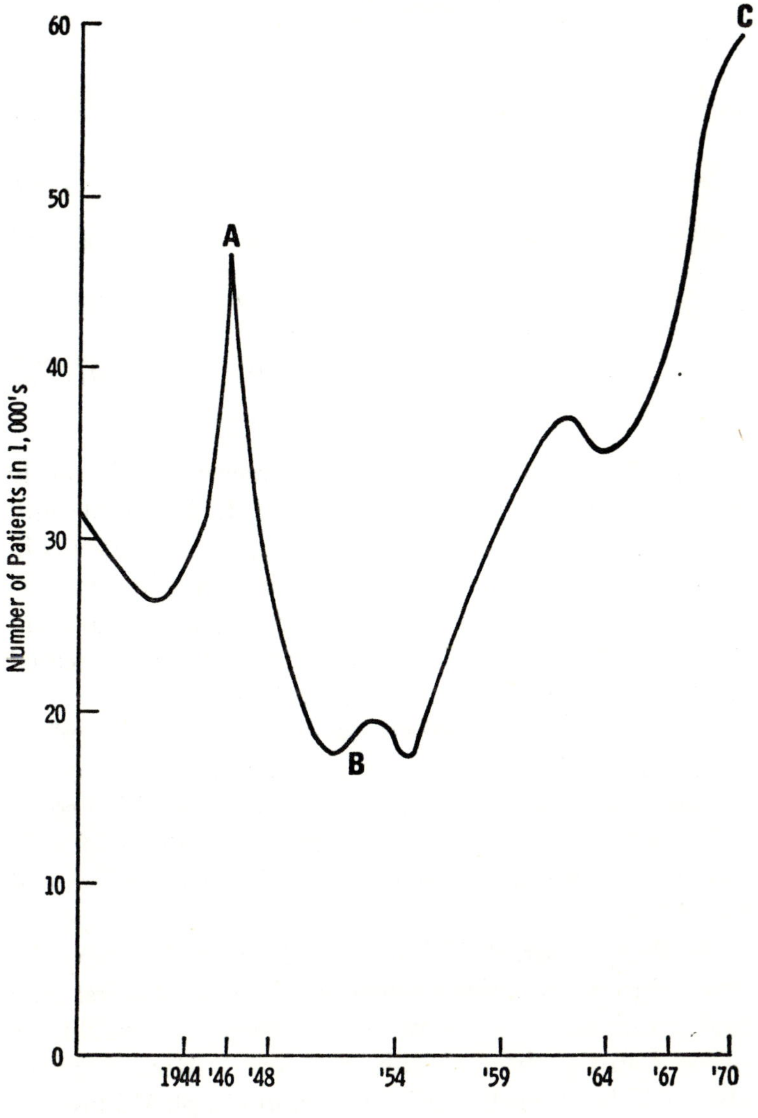

TABLE II

NON-GONOCOCCAL URETHRITIS

1952	11,552	1962	22,494
1954	13,279	1964	27,521
1956	14,825	1966	30,462
1958	17,606	1968	35,721
1960	22,004	1970	47,292

The decline in syphilis already mentioned is nicely illustrated in Table III and Graph III. This table and graph include all cases of syphilis seen as new patients in each particular year studied. It is seen that in 1970 the total was of the order of three and a quarter thousand patients. Many of these patients may have been treated in the past and many are certainly not infectious.

It is the early infectious patients that have syphilis who command the greatest attention for the health of the community because they have active disease which could infect sexual partners. Fortunately, the number of such patients has similarly lessened over the years. More will be said of this later.

By sharp contrast, Table IV and Graph IV show the upward trend of patients attending clinic for the first time and requiring some form of treatment for conditions other than the three already mentioned. More detail of these will be given later. Table V and Graph V illustrate

GRAPH II

RISING INCIDENCE OF NON-GONOCOCCAL URETHRITIS

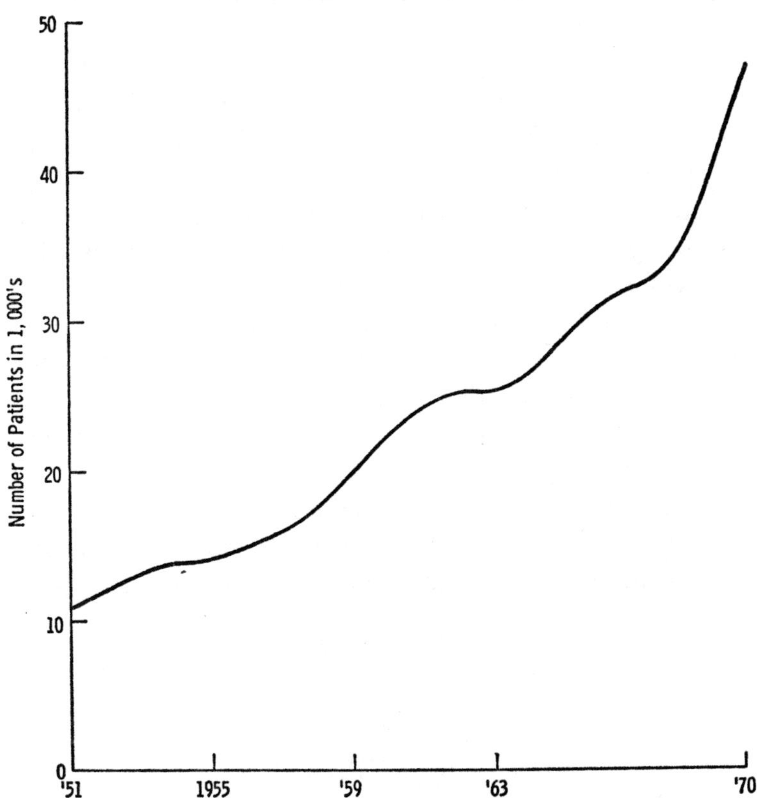

the large increase in those attending clinics but not requiring treatment. Each of these patients needs to be
entered into the register, interview, clinic examination,
certain tests and further follow-up interviews and reassurance of their good health. The time taken for this
process will be obvious. Indeed, Table VI and Graph VI
give an indication of the increased workload of special
treatment centres at the present time. In the past ten
years it has in fact, almost doubled. Why?

47

The increase in numbers of those affected by sexually transmitted disease is but one of the adverse social factors by which the disturbance of society may be measured today.

The denominators drugs, alcohol and suicide have already been compared. A comparison of our Graphs IV, V and VI and the second part of Graph I with the graph relating to drug use in Dr. Mitchell's manual on *Drugs* in this same Priory Care and Welfare Series gives an alarming lesson. The steeply accelerating rise of the last parts of each graph cannot escape notice.

Society finds itself, with its comparatively full employment and its luxuries, in a state of disturbed affluence, with insufficient outlet for its energies and aggressions. Under this aura of prosperous insecurity have developed escapes and defiances.

In the field of drugs the results are well known. In the sexual field, the social change takes the shape of increased sexual activity and experimentation of various sorts.

TABLE III

SYPHILIS

1952	7,122	1962	4,120
1954	5,281	1964	3,775
1956	5,141	1966	3,678
1958	4,326	1968	3,741
1960	3,946	1970	3,267

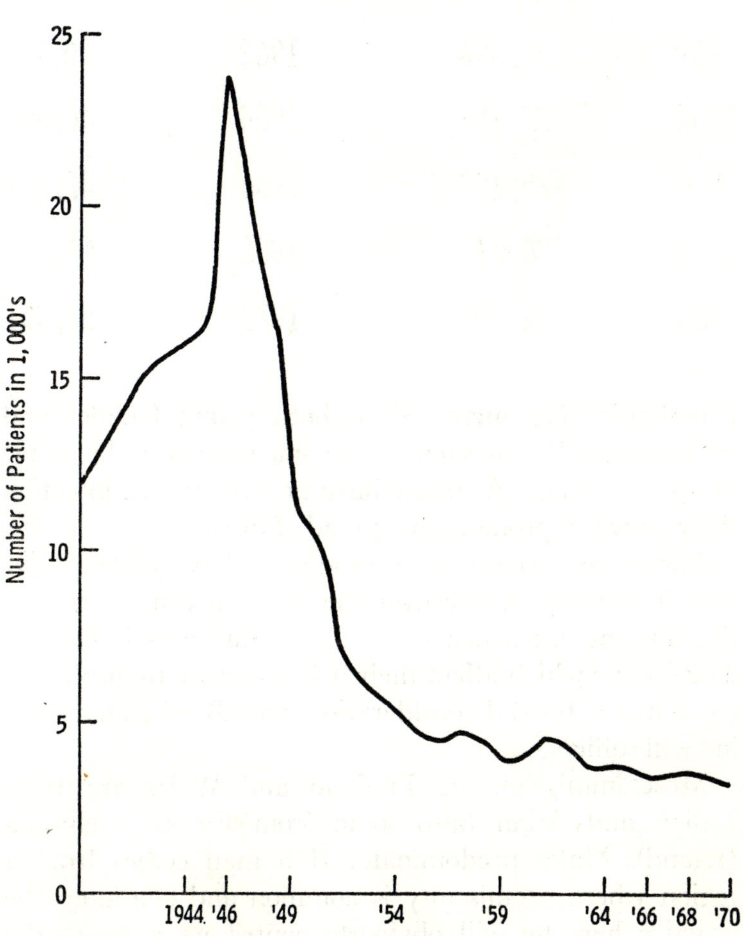
GRAPH III
DECLINING INCIDENCE OF SYPHILIS
25
20
15
10
5
0
Number of Patients in 1,000's
1944. '46   '49   '54   '59   '64 '66 '68 '70

TABLE IV

<u>REQUIRING TREATMENT</u>

1952	21,494	1962	36,217
1954	23,188	1964	40,122
1956	25,193	1966	47,697
1958	26,711	1968	61,667
1960	32,592	1970	87,351

Promiscuity has increased in both young females and young males. Females tend to become more sexually active at an earlier age. As many have no evidence of infection their activities promote the spread of disease.

Immigrants, coloured or otherwise, have played their part in varying degree over the years in contributing to the altering incidence of sexually transmitted diseases. The factors which affect their behaviour are multiple and too complex for full consideration here. Brief understanding will suffice.

Most immigrants to England and Wales are West Indian and Asian (also some from Europe including Ireland). Males predominate. If a man comes from a region where promiscuity is common and continues the practice here he will obviously contribute more to the increase of disease. Others away from their own country, families and friends may resort to sexual comfort as a substitute and as compensation for their insecurity.

GRAPH IV

OTHERS REQUIRING TREATMENT

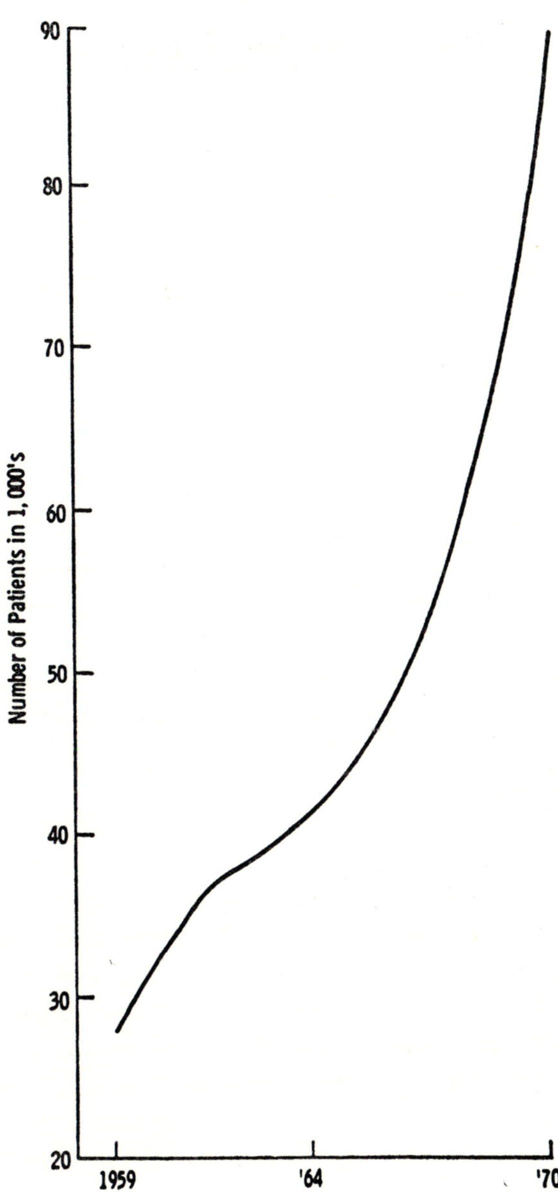

TABLE V

<u>NOT REQUIRING TREATMENT</u>

1952	37,488	1962	37,784
1954	34,154	1964	43,498
1956	32,349	1966	45,360
1958	30,712	1968	49,208
1960	36,963	1970	60,599

As an alternative to loneliness, sex is a bond which knows few social or racial barriers and needs no language. Since the early 1950s when the incidence of sexually transmitted diseases was low (see Graph I) immigrants caused increasing amounts of these diseases up to about 1960. By this time many were more settled. They were established in our community, had jobs secured; many had brought their wives and families over here or had a stable relationship with one woman.

Thus from 1960 onwards the influence of immigrants declined and they caused a lessening amount of sex disease whilst the home population of Britain caused more and more. More recently, it is the impression of some clinic doctors that the position of immigrants with regard to sexually transmitted disease is swinging back again. They seem now once again to be providing gradually increasing numbers of clinic-patients.

The reasons for this are not yet explained. Some immigrants may be getting over the social shock of coming

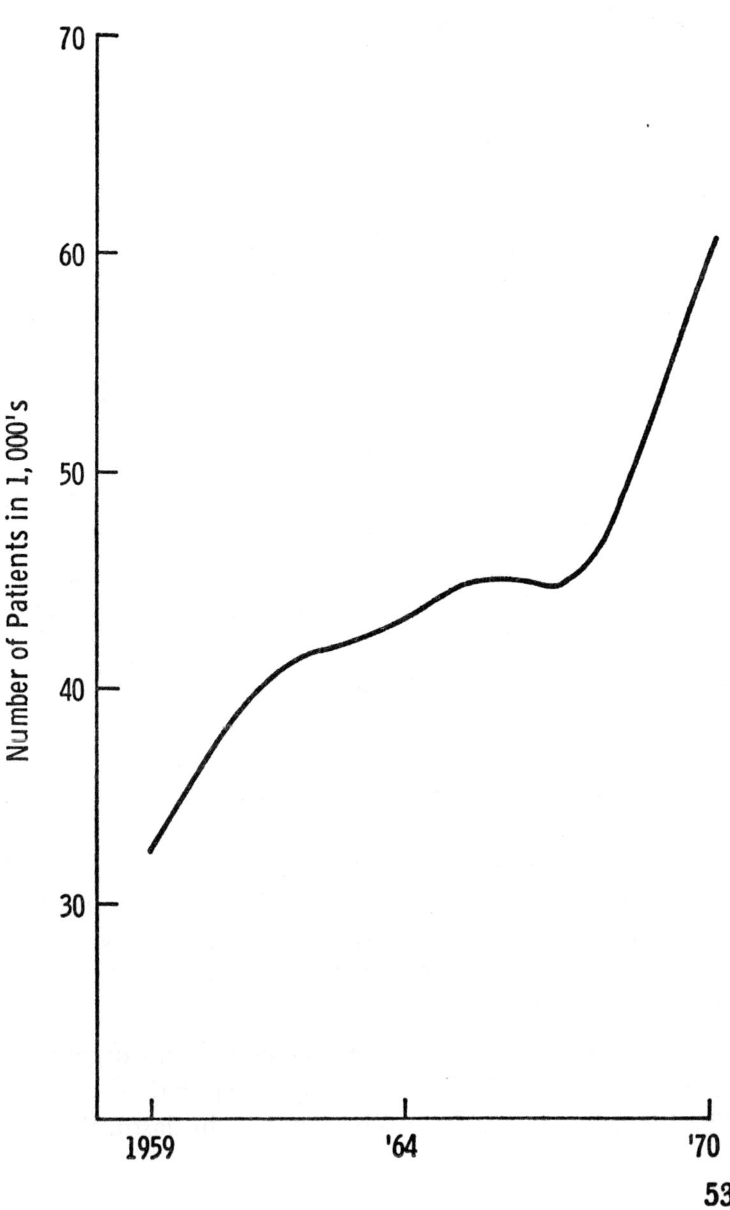
GRAPH V
OTHERS NOT REQUIRING TREATMENT
Number of Patients in 1,000's
70
60
50
40
30
1959
'64
'70

TABLE VI

TOTAL NEW PATIENTS. EXCLUDING CHANCROID

1952	96, 751	1962	138, 053
1954	93, 438	1964	152, 581
1956	97, 896	1966	164, 680
1958	107, 242	1968	195, 299
1960	129, 275	1970	253, 273

to live in another country and are now allowing themselves the same liberties as they knew in their own. Perhaps a new generation of immigrants born or largely brought up in this country is sexually integrated and behaving with the same sexual licence as the youth of our own population. For whatever complex reasons, the tendency is towards increasing disease.

There is evidence that prostitution as such is a declining practice. However, prostitutes of either sex still contribute considerably to the rising incidence of infections.

Increased population mobility also promotes spread of disease. A young person may acquire infection in one town and have casual sexual intercourse several times on the way to the next port of call. Not only does this spread disease territorially. As people on the move may not attend adequately for treatment, drug resistant organisms may be fostered. These cause further spread of disease. The itinerant she (or he) with sexual enthusiasm, thumb-

GRAPH VI

TOTAL NEW PATIENTS. EXCLUDING CHANCROID

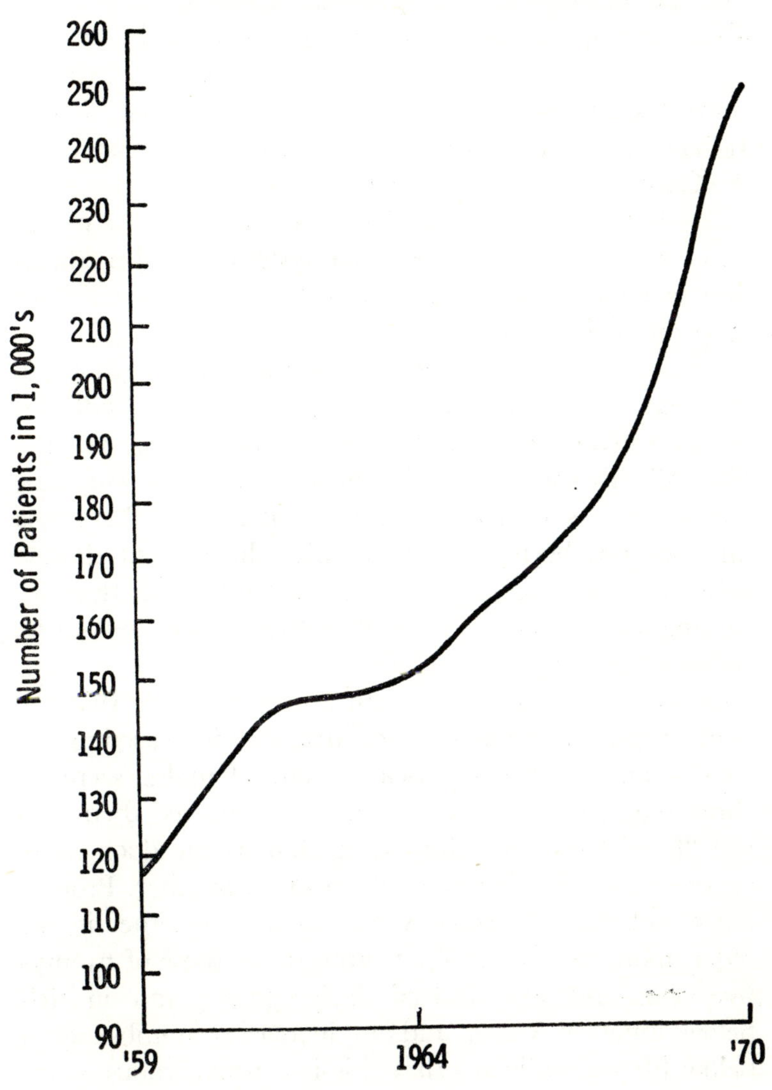

ing her way down our highways, by-ways and motorways has become a feature of modern travel. Beware infection!

Itinerant youth has, of course, lost the influence of the stability and control of home and parents. Indeed, it may be through lack of parental guidance and stable home atmosphere that the young person packs up and leaves. Whether by cause or effect, diminished parental control is associated with increased casual sex and disease. It has also been shown that the declining influence of the Church is similarly associated.

There has also been a lack of information to the public about sex and disease. The whole system of health education is under review and a much more comprehensive programme is foreseen.

During and after the last world war (1939-45/6) venereal diseases received huge publicity, especially on wayside advertisement hoardings, railway stations and the like. All this was swept aside in the face of the very low incidence of sexually transmitted diseases in the 1950s and has not been replaced despite the present disease crisis. Military conscription also ceased in 1960, thus depriving young males of sex education which used to be provided during National Service.

It seems likely from a recent American study that the contraceptive pill may be associated with increased promiscuity and increased disease. Some females seem to think that if the risk of pregnancy is removed then they are "freed" sexually—forgetting that as the door closes on one social disadvantage, it opens on another. Promiscuity and the pill probably only operate together in the older, more sophisticated age groups, *i.e.* those of twenty-five years and over. Indeed the pregnancy rate in girls below nineteen years, and an increasing number even below fifteen, indicates that this is a promiscuous sector

56

which seems to care little about protection against pregnancy.

That young people experiment sexually without due regard to the immediate or remote consequences is, perhaps, the root of the problem. Some may also be influenced by the attitudes and practices of some "trendy" figures in the entertainment world whose very wealth to some extent places them outside the limits of normal social behaviour. As their activities are widely glamourised in the mass entertainment and publicity media, their way of life is by some young people taken as a criterion. With all these influences, there grows the new conformity—"everyone's doing it, let's join in regardless."

Identifying the Diseases

I. GONORRHOEA

A typical clinical conversation:

DOCTOR: When was your last sexual intercourse?
PATIENT: Three days ago.
DOCTOR: Do you know the person?
PATIENT: Oh! yes. She's clean. She's my regular girl.
DOCTOR: How long have you known her?
PATIENT: Two weeks.
DOCTOR: In that time, you don't know her at all.

Gonorrhoea is a highly infectious disease which almost always starts in the genital organs. It is caused by a minute organism, a bacterium called the gonococcus. A related organism causes brain and spine inflammation, known as meningitis. Other related organisms live in the nose and throat and may at times cause inflammation in these areas. The gonococcus has become adapted to live in the genitals almost exclusively and is thus a cause of one type of sexually transmitted disease, namely gonorrhoea. So adapted has the bacterium become to the tissues in which it lives that, once outside the genital region, it usually dies rapidly.

Method of infection. It follows from the above that gonorrhoea is passed from one person to another, usually during sexual intercourse. Genital contact without actual entry of the penis into the vagina may also result in transmission of the infection, especially if either partner is losing considerable discharge. The same risk applies during rectal intercourse whether heterosexual or between homosexual males.

Transfer of infected discharge by hand contact from the genitals of one partner to the other is a fairly remote possibility. Mouth infection is rare, so mouth to mouth kissing is an unlikely method of transmission. Genital to mouth transfer is also a possibility. Cooking and eating utensils are not implicated; hardly, if ever, are lavatory seats, despite old wives' tales. The gonococcus is not adapted to live on lavatory seats. If a pregnant woman has untreated gonorrhoea, her child may get serious eye infection during birth. The infection, is, however, treatable.

A patient with gonorrhoea may, by hand, transfer infection from genitals to eyes. Infants and young girls may get genital infection either from contact with an infected parent, e.g. playing in bed, or from towels used in simultaneous toilet with an infected person.

Symptoms and signs. "Incubation" is the interval between the infecting intercourse and the time when the disease could be shown to be present by examination and tests. For gonorrhoea, this interval is about two to four days in both males and females. At this time, many men will begin to notice their infection although some take longer—even up to two or three weeks. Women, however, are unlikely to be aware of the infection at this early stage.

For patients to seek help, they must either be suspicious of their consort or they must actually notice that something is abnormal. In the female, no abnormal indications may be noticed for weeks or even months. (The same delay may apply in the rectally infected homosexual.) The disease may be accelerated, or brought to a girl's notice, by her first menstrual period after infection.

A symptom one feels, a sign one sees.

The main *symptom* of gonoccocal genital infection in the male is dysuria (discomfort or pain, chiefly when passing urine). The amount of this discomfort depends on how easily the patient feels pain. Some deny any appreciable disturbance. Others complain bitterly, "as if I were passing razor blades". While the sensation is usually felt most during the passage of urine, some patients seem to feel more discomfort just *after*; others complain of discomfort all the time.

The main *sign* of gonorrhoea in the male is discharge from the opening of the urine passage at the tip of the penis. This discharge is usually green or yellow and may be blood-stained. The amount varies from patient to patient. However, it is usually obvious and quite distinct from the normal glossy moisture which is seen if the lips of the urethral opening are parted with the fingers.

In many cases the discharge is profuse and runs on to the underwear or trousers causing crusted stains and leading to much discomfort. These are not to be confused with the coloured stains, yellowish-brown on underwear, which are not crusted and cannot be detected by touch. These are urine stains due to dribbling of the last drops of urine after emptying the bladder and are normal.

A further complaint may be of over frequent passage of small amounts of urine. This is termed urinary frequency and is less common in males than females.

At this stage, the infection is of short duration, is localised in the front or anterior urethra and will in all

60

likelihood be free of complications. This is when most sensible men will at once go to a clinic. It is of very great importance not to delay as this may lead to spread of the infection and complicated disease. Delay also means that the tracing of contacts is deferred and this in its turn may cause spread of infection in the woman or women con-

URETHRAL DISCHARGE

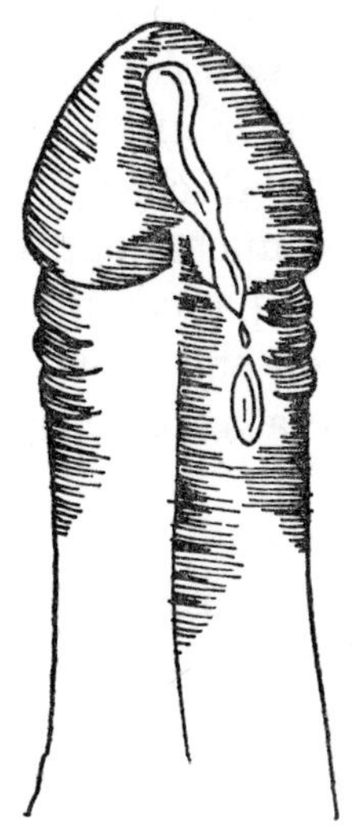

Figure 5

cerned, to say nothing of any men with whom they have intercourse before they are treated.

At the clinic, a history of the disease is recorded, note being made of any complicating feature. Particular regard is given to the sexual history, the dates of any recent sexual intercourse being noted. It is important to determine as far as is possible the infecting intercourse and to be quite sure whether the patient has had further intercourse since that time with a different woman, or man, or both. (The wary physician recognises that in the present sexually variegated society all manner of sexual relations are encountered and he casts his diagnostic net widely.)

All patients are seen individually by the doctor. A brief general medical check-up is ideally performed on each patient. In particular the genital and anal areas are examined and samples of the urethral discharge taken with a sterile loop of platinum wire or a sterile cotton wool swab. From these samples microscope slides are made and stained by special methods which show any gono-coccus present in the discharge. This examination of the stained slide by microscope enables the diagnosis to be made whilst the patient is there in the clinic and treatment provided on the spot—an important part in the control of such a rapidly spreading infection as gonorrhoea.

While the microscope slides are being prepared examination for other possible infections is made, for example, *trichomonas vaginalis* (see later). A cotton wool swab of the discharge is also sent to the public health laboratory along with one of the slides smeared with discharge. The laboratory can thus examine the slide and confirm or deny the diagnosis made in the clinic. Still further proof is provided by culturing the swab on special jelly in low temperature ovens. All this is satisfying sup-port that the diagnosis and treatment in the clinic were correct. It may also assume great importance if produced in court of law. Divorce proceedings on grounds of marital infidelity are not uncommon sequels to gonococcal in-fection.

A sample of blood is taken routinely on all patients and sent to the blood department of the public health laboratory. A group of tests for syphilis is performed. As syphilis may develop many weeks after the patient first attends clinic, it is common sense that the blood test must be repeated at the end of his follow up programme to make sure that it has not become positive for syphilis.

In the clinic the microscope slides will have been prepared and the patient is then asked to pass a certain amount of urine into the first of two glass jars, and a further amount, if he can, in the second. (If you are visiting a clinic for a check it is well to remember not to pass urine for at least an hour before so that you can provide these samples.) As many people have psychological difficulty in urinating in disturbed surroundings, privacy is provided for this procedure. The first sample is cloudy with pus from the discharge. Providing the second urine is clear, the inferrence is that the infection is confined to the front of the urethra and that complications are unlikely. Clouding of the second sample denotes extension of the infection. Further tests and additional treatment will probably be needed.

The case assessed and proper treatment provided, the patient is told to return in one week for tests to show that the discharge has been cured and the urine cleared. The rest of the follow-up programme is arranged, but —as I said earlier—a patient should not need to attend more than a few times in all.

Before leaving the clinic after treatment, the patient is given a contact card bearing his number and the diagnosis in code. This he must give to "the infecting consort," i.e. the person he got the disease from. Another contact card is provided if he admits to intercourse with another person after having become infected. *This method of seeking out infected women to attend clinic is one of the most valuable measures in attempting to control this disease.* It is of first importance that the doctors and nurses foster a sufficient relationship with the patient that he agrees to try and fulfil this duty of contact tracing.

If the "contact" presents the card on attendance then the clinic know that that particular search has been successful and the person is saved a lot of questions being asked. As there is a coded diagnosis on this card the clinic staff know exactly what to look for. Failing this, a description of the infecting person and her address may be obtained and given to a health visitor (a nurse with special training—see later) who will then go and find the infected person and get her to attend. If her address is fully known, letters may be sent inviting her to attend.

However, arranging a visit is often time consuming and both visiting and letter-delivery may embarrass some people and it is therefore far better from all points of view if she responds to the presentation of the contact slip and brings it to the clinic. I can hardly over-stress the fact that the control of gonorrhoea has as much to do with detection as it has to do with medicine. Detection requires team-work and the team includes the patients.

Complications. Patients should attend clinic early, as soon as they note anything amiss. Delay may lead to complicated infection.

Infection in the male may be limited to the front part of the urethra lying below the prostate gland. If neglected, it may spread to the back part of the urethra and to other structures. Obviously, the doctor's assessment of the patient's illness is assisted if he can decide whether the infection is only in the front urethra or whether it has spread to the back as well. It is to help this diagnosis that men are asked to pass two urine samples (see page

63) after tests have been made on the urethral discharge.

If infection of the front urethra spreads it may involve small glands at each side of the urethral opening. They may become red, swollen, shiny and painful and sometimes drops of pus can be seen on each. Alongside the urethra, in the body or shaft of the penis, run several channels parallel with the urethra and connected to it at intervals by small tubes or ducts. The infection may spread to any of these tubes and channels. This may cause discomfort, pain or tenderness in the penis. The infection may become localised to form a sort of boil inside the penis and this can be extremely painful.

Tender and painful lumps may appear in the groins showing that the infection is affecting the glands in the groins.

The large veins which run the length of the top-side of the penis may become affected. The inflammation sometimes causes clotting (thrombosis) of the blood in these veins. This blocks the veins so that the blood and fluid of the circulation cannot flow out of the penis as it should, so the penis becomes painful and very swollen. The swollen penis is so waterlogged that pressure and friction of the clothing may rub away the surface of the skin so that ulcers are formed. As these may become infected by other bacteria the situation goes from bad to worse. Sometimes a gland under the skin behind the scrotum becomes inflamed and swollen. This can cause pain deep in the pelvis, perhaps associated with sitting and on bowel emptying. It may also cause some leakage of fluid from the urethral opening.

Infection spreading to the back urethra which connects the bladder to the prostate gland may cause inflammation of the prostate itself and possibly affect several other important structures.

3—VDE * *

V.D. Explained

In the scrotum are the two testicles. Each testicle produces a chemical or hormone (which affects the maleness of the individual) and sperms. These collect in a "depot" called the epididymis behind each testicle. There are two sperm-fluid glands (seminal vesicles) behind a man's urinary bladder. These form fluid for the sperms from the testicles to float in. The tube from the sperm "depot" joins the tube from the sperm-fluid glands and they all meet the urethra as it passes through the prostate gland. The prostate also has its own tubes opening into the urethra. When a man reaches sexual climax the sperm-depots, the sperm fluid glands and the prostate gland all squeeze their contents down their tubes into the urethra and the milky fluid comes from the opening of the urethra at the end of the penis.

If the infection of gonorrhoea spreads from the back urethra the sperm "depot" may become very sore, swollen and painful. The testicle on that side may be affected, fluid collects and it becomes swollen. After the condition subsides, the tube from the "depot" may be blocked in more or less degree. The blockage can be complete and permanent. If this happens on both sides the man will no longer be able to contribute any sperms in a sexual relationship. This means that he will not be able to make a baby with his chosen sex partner. He is called sterile.

If the sperm fluid gland is affected the patient may experience deep pelvic pains and gland fluids and perhaps blood may run from the urethral opening.

If the prostate gland is involved by the spreading infection, the illness may be acute (short-time) or chronic (long-time). In acute inflammation, the patient is often feverish with pelvic pain and other serious painful disturbance of bowel and bladder function. He may not be able to pass urine at all. Chronic prostatic involvement is uncommon and may not be associated with much pain but there is often persistent urethral discharge and the patient may become neurotic.

Complications affecting other than the sexual and pelvic organs may occur due to infection spreading through the blood stream. This will normally only happen after the disease has been present untreated, or inadequatedly treated, for several weeks or longer and is therefore not common.

Arthritis is the blood-carried complication most often seen. It is said to be more common in women but this is not proved. Skin infection may co-exist. Other blood-borne complications remote from the pelvis have been described and affect the heart, the spine and brain and cause one form of eye inflammation. These are hardly, if ever, seen nowadays due to the development of diagnostic and treatment services and no doubt also due to the generally increased standard of living and nutrition.

The eye is definitely at risk in gonococcal infection but not as a blood spread disease. More will be said of this later.

Finally, it must be realised that where treatment has been delayed or inadequate, the male patient may suffer scarring of the urethra. Scar tissue contracts as time goes by and this may lessen the diameter of the urethra. In later years this may interfere with the patient's ability to empty his bladder and he may require instruments to be passed up his penis to relieve him of urine. Sometimes a surgical operation may be performed on the urethra to take away the narrow part and to try and make a better, wider urethra. However, the results are often less than hoped for and not many surgeons are eager to undertake the task.

Gonorrhoea in the female. Male patients often say that the women concerned have no symptoms or signs and feel perfectly well and will not attend. We ask male patients to stress to the women who are their sources of infection that they *are* ill, although they feel well.

Two contacts are often involved. The infection comes *from* the primary contact and is given *to* the secondary contact. The primary contact is often a casual acquaintance and is best sought initially by contact slip. If this method fails the auxiliary helpers are used.

In large clinics social workers are available and the Department of Health is eager to promote more people to work in this field. Ideally, two full-time Welfare Officers share the work which falls into two categories, namely (a) Interview and (b) Search. The male patient is *interviewed* and all the information about the primary contact obtained. This is passed to the second Welfare Officer who then *searches* for the contact. If there is no answer after repeated visits at a given address, a written message can be left with instructions to attend a clinic. Further visits and letters may follow.

The secondary contact is often the wife or regular girlfriend of the patient, and he is asked to bring her to the clinic. If he is unwilling or unsuccessful a specially trained nurse (health visitor) can be asked to help. The situation is emotionally charged and requires delicate handling.

As mentioned, the outcome of untreated infection in the *male* is toward eventual diminishing symptoms and signs with or without associated damage. The infection either "dies out" or at least becomes hidden in which case the man is a carrier. In the *female*, the infection gradually progresses and vaginal discharge makes its appearance. Many women have a certain amount of

68

vaginal discharge as a normal feature of their lives. Any *alteration* of discharge which then comes to notice should prompt her to seek proper advice. The infected female will probably also complain of some urinary discomfort but this is a far less constant feature than it is in the male.

Additional local complaints are usually secondary to the vaginal discharge and inflammation. At a minimum there may be vague irritation or discomfort at the vaginal entrance. At worst there is copious, pouring vaginal discharge with violent inflammation of the vagina and neighbouring skin even extending on to the lower abdomen, the groins and upper thighs. Discharge tracks backwards, especially when the woman lies on her back at night and sometimes severe inflammation of the anus and rectum results. Secondary ulceration and bacterial infection of the inflamed skin may occur. Sitting and walking may be painful. The primary sites of infection are the canal which runs through the neck of the womb and the urethra. In the absence of treatment, complications occur.

Complications. Spread of infection to structures surrounding the urethra, similar to that occurring in the male, may occur. The principal complications are infection of the glands at either side of the urethral opening. Again, swollen red apertures may be seen with pus in each. Glands in the large folds of skin which surround the urethral and vaginal openings may also become inflamed. This usually happens on one side rather than both and causes a swelling. The woman may be feverish, and the swelling—which may reach the size of a tennis-ball—is so painful that any movement becomes almost impossible. The groin glands may be enlarged, tender and painful.

From the lining of the canal in the neck of the womb (the canal of the cervix or cervical canal) infection may spread up past the lining of the womb itself.

The monthly periods may be disturbed and this, in a woman who is usually quite "regular" may be a first sign. Infection spreading to structures alongside the womb may cause abscess, with pelvic pain or discomfort. Further spread can involve the tubes which connect the womb to the ovaries which produce the female's eggs. An abscess may form in one or other of these tubes, sometimes both.

The symptoms and signs are not easy to diagnose and often appear rather like appendicitis. If the family doctor is called in, he is not likely to be given the patient's sex history and he will probably call the surgeon. Patients may be operated on and the true condition is only then found. Further complication may occur if abscess forms around an ovary. This may go on to produce more or less inflammation of the lining of the pelvis and lower abdomen—peritonitis.

It is important that women at sex-risk should take note of any pelvic and low-abdominal pain and of any period disturbance and should seek proper advice.

The eye. Sexual partners may by hand transfer gonococcal pus from their own genitals, or from their partner, to their own eyes or those of their partner. In such cases the organism grows on the front membrane of the eye and produces a discharge. The sight may be threatened if prompt treatment is not provided.

Further, where a child is born to a woman who has untreated gonococcal infection, the baby's eyes may well become infected during its escape down the infected birth passage during confinement. This is one form of

70

"sticky-eye" after birth and such an eye should always be tested to see just which bacterium is causing the trouble. Where gonorrhoea is present, severe eye damage, even resulting in complete blindness, may well result if the child is not properly treated.

The mother with gonorrhoea will also need treatment at once, and contacts must be sought.

Children. Modes of living, like fashions, change. Sexually achieved urethral gonorrhea has been reported in a boy of only six. However, in very young girls, genital gonorrhoea can be acquired accidentally, especially if they are in the habit of visiting their elders in bed in the morning. A young girl bouncing around on an infected adult may well pick up some of the infected discharge and get an infection of the juvenile vulva. They may complain little or not at all but parents may notice them scratching between their legs. The child may have difficulty in walking because of soreness of the skin around the groins. She may cry every time she passes urine because it causes so much smarting. A parent may notice the inflamed skin at the top of the thighs and between the legs. Similar chance transference of gonorrhoea to young girls by infected towels and clothing are considered a possibility.

Where gonorrhoea is found in the young of either sex, the situation is often emotionally highly charged and its handling requires skill. The question of criminal interference with the child is always present.

The homosexual. The male homosexual is often very promiscuous and so plays a considerable part in promoting the spread of gonorrhoea. Some use their penis in the sex act and are often called the "active" partner.

Some offer their rectum and are called the "passive" partner. Many play both roles. Some who use the penis go indiscriminately with both men and women.

The female homosexual features much less in sexually transmitted diseases. This is expected, as it is the male penis which transfers disease from one person to the next in nearly all cases.

Gonorrhoea of the urethra in the homosexual male is the same as in heterosexuals. In the rectum, the disease is comparable to gonorrhoea in the female, and the passive patient often has to be sent to the clinic by someone he has infected. There may be no symptoms or signs at all. These may develop weeks after his rectum has become infected but by this time he may have passed the disease to many others.

Symptoms include anal itching, soreness or discomfort. Some leakage from the anus is usual at some stage. It may be slight mucus (like thin slime or saliva) or thicker matter. It can be so marked as to wet the clothing through. Sometimes there is bleeding. If the discharge is marked, the skin round the anus and the touching sides of the buttocks soon gets sore and cracked and can be very painful. The patient often feels the need to empty his bowel all the time, even though he has just done so.

"Invisible" gonorrhoea. Unrecognised early gonorrhoea in the female and in the male rectum have been mentioned. Two further situations of unsuspected infection should be understood:

1. In some males there is no recognised discharge or burning sensation. Such men can be said to be gonorrhoea carriers and are able to infect other people.

2. Although most women tend to get symptoms and signs which would eventually cause them to seek clinical advice, some go through the early stages with only moderate disturbance, the complications described above do not happen, and the infection settles down to a low-grade chronic state.

Such a woman may feel a bit "off-colour" but she complains of no special symptoms or signs. Her last sex experience may be months previously, yet she is infective and a man having unprotected sexual intercourse with her is liable to catch gonorrhoea.

It follows from these considerations about "invisible" gonorrhoea, that where a person has been at risk and there is a chance that a contact has infection, then the person should attend clinic for a thorough check-up. A contact may have a contact-card issued by a clinic to hand to the unsuspecting person: this should be taken to a convenient clinic without delay. Alternatively, the suggestion may be verbal and it may not even be at first hand. "Jack says you've given him V.D. You're to go to a clinic. He won't speak to you himself." If there are no symptoms or signs, the person to whom this sort of thing is said is in a dilemma. It is one of the oldest sick jokes to hint that someone has some form of sexually transmitted disease. The "accused" person may suffer anxiety for months before seeking advice. The best course of action is obvious—just in case there is some infection, and to save all that doubt and distress, go and find out straightaway.

Diagnosis and treatment. Samples of discharge or secretion are taken from the urethra in the male and from the urethra and cervical canal in the female. Rectal

73

samples are taken in certain instances, and samples are taken from the vagina for other investigations.

Smears on glass slides are made from the urethral and cervical specimens and cultures are prepared for the laboratory. In the clinic, the smears are stained and examined by microscope, a diagnosis made and the treatment given. This usually is one or two injections only. In men, if the two-glass urine test indicates spread of infection, or if there are clinically obvious complications, further treatment will be provided. The standard treatment is Penicillin, but if a patient has a known allergy to this drug, other treatments are available. The patient should not have sexual intercourse, or drink alcohol, until the disease has been cured. Both act as irritants to an already inflamed urethra and it is only common sense to let an injured part of the body settle down before again subjecting it to stresses and strains. If you pull a muscle in your leg at football, you don't go out and play another game—you rest it!

2. NON-SPECIFIC URETHRITIS

Some short statements may make this difficult disease situation more understandable:

(*a*)   Urethritis may due to gonorrhoea. If it is not, it can be called non-gonococcal urethritis.

(*b*)   Non-gonoccocal urethritis can be due to different known causes, e.g. fungus infection, a small organism called *Trichomonas vaginalis,* bladder infection, etc. There may have been old infection or injury leading to urethral narrowing, instruments and chemicals may have been introduced by the patient for sexual experience or for fear of sex disease. There could be a generalised

74

disease such as diabetes. Warts in the urethra can cause a discharge. Syphilis in the urethra, cancer, tuberculosis are rare possibilities but ones which the doctor must consider, and, it is hoped, exclude.

When known causes are excluded, regretfully one is left with a urethritis for which no specific cause can be found—hence the name non-specific urethritis (N.S.U. for short). This situation, with inflammation usually confined to the urethra, is a condition suffered almost exclusively by males. The difference in length between the male and female urethra makes it unlikely that there would be any strictly comparable disease in women. They do sometimes get a non-specific genital or pelvic infection, they are prone to cystitis, and may also suffer chronic infection of the neck of the womb (cervicitis). Just what connection any or each of these conditions has with N.S.U. is not known.

The cause of N.S.U. is unknown and until that has been clarified its relation to any disease in women cannot be definitely stated. The length of time between infection and symptoms is so variable that there may be more than one cause. It seems likely that a virus is responsible and it could be that different strains of virus have different incubation periods. One thing which does seem established is the connection of the disease with sexual intercourse. If patients' stories are true, a few cases seem to happen without any sex experience. In such circumstances it may be that the infection occurs in a urethra damaged in some way, e.g. sports injury. Some cases occur when a young man has intercourse for the first time or begins to have regular sex experience.

A similar situation obtains where a man has been apart from his wife or regular partner for a time and then recommences intercourse with her, extra-marital relations being denied by both partners. In other instances the man suffers urethritis if he has consistently used a contraceptive sheath for a while and then has sexual intercourse with the same woman but without a sheath. It apparently occurs also in some men who always use a sheath. It should be remembered though that many men use a sheath only for the climax of the sex act which, as far as infection is concerned, is equivalent to not using a sheath at all. Other cases occur where a man has a regular sex partner but has intercourse once with a different woman.

N.S.U. also apparently occurs in the male when neither partner admits sexual intercourse with anyone else. In some of these cases there is a history that the woman has recently started taking a contraceptive pill or has recently changed from one brand to another. Just what relation, if any, the pill has to N.S.U. is not clear. In any event, the N.S.U. is believed to be infective in origin and it must be borne in mind that the sex-history of either partner may not be accurate.

It will be understood that where a man is very promiscuous and repeatedly has several different sex partners, then it will be impossible to say just from whom he contracted the infection. The disease can also be contracted homosexually.

From what has been said you will see that medical knowledge on the above condition is far from complete and is mainly held up because the cause, or causes, of the condition is unknown. However, a summary of the general principles may be made:

(*a*)   N.S.U. mainly affects males.
(*b*)   The cause is not known.

(*c*)   It may be due to a virus which may also cause some eye disease.

(*d*)   It is often associated with an occasion of sexual intercourse with a partner the man is not used to.

(*e*)   It usually does no harm.

(*f*)   It does not carry the same implication as gonorrhoea. Gonorrhoea cannot occur if two sex partners "stick to" each other and don't have sex with anyone else. N.S.U. apparently can happen between regular partners.

Symptoms and signs. After a variable length of time following the infecting intercourse, the man begins to get the symptoms and signs of urethritis—urethral discharge and abnormal sensation on passing urine. The symptoms and signs may appear two or three days after the sex exposure which is thought to be the infecting one or it may take several weeks to develop. Commonly the incubation period is two to four weeks, and there is great variation in the amount of trouble each patient experiences. The urinary discomfort is so slight in some patients that they hesitate to say that it is present at all. Some, indeed, deny its existence. The discharge also may be so scanty that it is not seen on the patient's first visit to the clinic.

In these circumstances an attempt may be made to obtain a sample of discharge by scraping the urethra with a platinum wire and smearing the result on a glass slide for the microscope. Alternatively, the patient can be asked if he will limit his intake of fluids that night so that he can attend clinic again first thing the following morning without having passed urine at home on waking. The doctor can then see what discharge has collected during the night. Many patients do attend clinic claiming that they only see discharge first thing in the morning. It is essential that the clinic staff see this and take samples for diagnosis, so that proper treatment can be given. At the other end of the scale some patients with N.S.U. have so much discomfort that they are afraid of passing urine and the discharge is so mattery, green and plentiful that the clinical picture certainly suggests gonorrhoea.

Between these extremes, most men with N.S.U. have slight or moderate pain when passing urine and moderate yellowish, rather watery discharge which is often slimy or sticky to the touch. The sides of the urethral opening may, in fact, be stuck together by it and the small amount of dried discharge round the opening forms yellowish-brown flakes or crusts. At this stage patients usually attend clinic for help.

Treatment. In uncomplicated cases, microscope slides are smeared for examination at the clinic and laboratory and a urethral culture also sent to the laboratory. A wet specimen in salt solution should also be examined on a different type of microscope to make sure no cause is being missed, for instance, Trichomonas and Thrush (see later). Routine blood tests are taken, as on all patients newly attending, to be sure that no syphilis is present. No gonorrhoea or other cause being found, the diagnosis is N.S.U. and routine treatment prescribed.

The treatment usually involves the patient taking a tablet four times a day for seven days and drinking plenty of fluids, except alcohol. This routine settles the infection in up to nine out of ten patients and more of the tablets, or a course of different treatment, can be provided if it does not. Larger doses for longer periods may be given.

A follow-up programme is arranged so that the infection can be declared cured. The patient is told when to return for check-up and blood tests for final exclusion of syphilis are repeated three months after the infecting intercourse, the patient usually needing to attend only four or five times in all during that time.

Although the cause of N.S.U. is not properly understood, it seems common sense to see the infecting partner. She will be given specific treatment even though, as explained, examination and tests on her will probably show nothing definite. Thus whatever the infection is, then it has been treated in both partners and with the same treatment which was effective in the man.

Men treated for N.S.U. may well never have any further trouble, but it is a recurrent condition and it cannot be guaranteed that a further attack will not occur. It may be that he will get a further attack if he has sex with a different partner, or if he has sex under altered conditions, e.g. with his wife when she is pregnant or with his regular partner when she is menstruating. And, if the patient's story is true, N.S.U. can recur without any further sexual exposure at all. The processes of diagnosis and treatment are provided as described, but no satisfactory explanation can be given.

Many patients may have several attacks over a period of weeks or months and need considerable mental support in addition to routine treatment. They should realise that in time they appear to develop resistance to attacks, the recurrences cease and there is no evidence that any permanent damage has been suffered. It is true, however, that where attacks are unduly persistent, further investigation for complications is necessary. A bladder infection may be suspected. Treatment and search for a cause will be necessary. Instruments and x-ray examinations may show some abnormality of the kidney, bladder or genital passages.

Some patients get pain and swelling of the testicle when the sperm "depot" (epididymis) becomes infected. In others, the prostate may be affected and it seems probable that prostatitis may be the cause of some patients' illness. In some, again, prostatic inflammation may be associated with back-ache and stiffening of the joints of the pelvis and lower spine.

Uncommonly, about one in every 100 patients with N.S.U. develop a generalised illness affecting many tissues of the body. This is usually called Reiter's disease. In addition to the urethritis, the end of the penis may peel and become very sore and the skin in various parts of the body may show degrees of inflammation, especially on the feet. The eyes and mouth are often sore and some joints swell with arthritis which can be quite severe. Such a condition, it can be imagined, needs much care and various treatments according to the areas of the body affected. It may be in the patient's best interest if he goes into hospital for a time, especially to allow proper care of joints.

Nearly all these patients eventually get back to normal strength and work again, but—just as with N.S.U.— further attack is a possibility against which there is no guarantee.

To sum up, N.S.U. is an ill-understood condition which costs many man-hours to patients and clinic staff. It is usually more of a nuisance than damaging but is occasionally associated with significant general ill-health.

3. SYPHILIS

This disease is caused by a spiral organism called a *Treponeme*. There are various organisms in this group: some live in animals; some live in man, perhaps in the gums around the teeth and apparently do no harm. The particular type we are interested in here is called *Treponema pallidum.* It may cause non-sexual syphilis in some populations in other countries. Closely related organisms may cause other non-sexual disease in some parts of the world. The blood of patients so affected may show positive tests for syphilis. For example, youngsters in the West Indies may get a disease called Yaws caused by the *Treponema pertenue.* The main trouble at first is big sores on the legs. As children touch and knock against each other, the leg sores can pass from one child to the next.

In syphilis, the *Treponema pallidum* (a whitish, spiral organism which looks like a corkscrew) nearly always causes a genital sore and the physical contact which passes the disease from one person to another is thus nearly always sexual.

The offending organism is microscopic in size—usually measured in millionths of a metre. About two thousand of them end to end would measure only $2\frac{1}{2}$ centimetres (or about an inch). The organism is so narrow it has almost no width at all. Down a microscope with special lighting it is seen to be alive, bending and jerking about. It multiplies by splitting across the middle and both ends go on living and growing like a worm cut in two. In this way it can rapidly form enormous numbers once it gets into the body.

A syphilitic patient may remain infectious for about two years after becoming infected. Certainly four years after infection he is most unlikely to pass infection to a sex partner. Thus, although every untreated case of syphilis is a matter of medical importance, the special treatment of early infectious cases is a matter of priority. Such patients must be diagnosed and treated quickly and their sex partners found equally quickly. In this way the disease can soon be halted in the patient and prevented from doing further damage. The health of the general public is also protected as the treated patient will no longer be able to pass the infection on to anyone.

Table III and Graph III earlier in the book show the fall in the total known new cases of syphilis at all stages. Although there have been notable outbreaks in recent times, especially in large cities, the incidence of new infectious cases has generally shown the same downward trend.

The number of new cases of primary, secondary and early latent syphilis reported in 1970 in England and Wales was, in fact, only 1,583. Compared with the 54,764 cases of gonorrhoea the incidence of syphilis seems unimportant. But for centuries this disease has been a killer —and were it not for Penicillin, improved diagnosis and energetic follow-up and contact tracing, it still would be. It seems unlikely that it will again become so common and deadly as previously but we cannot adopt a complacent attitude towards syphilis.

Syphilis may be *acquired*, i.e. caught from someone by contact, usually sexual, or *congenital*, i.e. caught by baby whilst still in the womb of a mother infected by syphilis.

Acquired syphilis. This disease is usually passed from sexual organs, or nearby, to a corresponding site in the sexual partner.

Occasionally, the infection may start at the corner of the mouth or on the lip surface. Such infection is caught by kissing a person with syphilis of the mouth or by mouth-genital contact. Accidental infection of the hands is a remote possibility in dentists, nurses and doctors attending syphilitic patients. Care in handling, use of protective gloves and frequent hand washing should prevent such an accident.

The disease is conventionally divided into stages:

Early
(a)   First stage or primary
(b)   Second stage or secondary
(c)   Early latent

Late
(a)   Late latent
(b)   Third stage, or tertiary
(c)   Fourth stage, or quarternary.

These stages may merge and overlap. The incubation period from infection to appearance of disease can be anything from nine to ninety days. It is often about three or four weeks.

Primary syphilis. Following infection and the incubation period, the presence of disease is demonstrated by the appearance of a spot at the site of the original infection. This spot soon loses its top and becomes a sore which may be so small that it is not noticed or as big as a $\frac{1}{2}$p coin. In most cases, quite a lot of inflammatory swelling surrounds the sore so that it feels quite hard if pressed with the fingers. It has been described as feeling like a button submerged in the skin. It often looks much worse than it feels, and frequently there is little pain. This is not a reliable diagnostic feature, however, since the sores can be painful and tender to handle.

The sore is usually single but if in contact with another skin surface, it can spread to that surface and form another sore. For example, if the sore is on the underside of the penis at or near the fraenum (the string-like structure which connects the foreskin to the underside of the penis) it could spread on to the front surface of the scrotum. More or less circular in shape, the lesion usually has a definite edge, a flat reddish stringy base and if knocked or squeezed is more likely to "weep" a little colourless fluid than actually bleed.

SYPHILITIC SORE

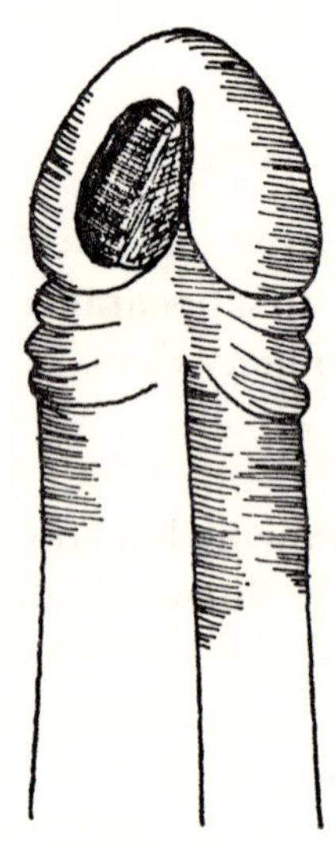

Figure 6

In the heterosexual male, the sore is almost always on the genitals. The usual place on the penis is the coronal sulcus. Another common area is near the fraenum, or it may be on the foreskin itself, either on the outside or inside, and it may be just a small crack-like area on the free border of the skin.

Other areas in which the sore occurs are on the glans; at the urethral opening or actually inside the opening—

making it rather difficult to find; on the shaft of the penis, on the scrotum or in the pubic hair—a situation which is more likely if the rest of the penis has been protected by a rubber sheath contraceptive.

In the female, the sore is commonly on the folds of skin which border the vaginal opening, the labia. Because of the looseness of the labia and surrounding tissues, a lot of inflammatory fluid may collect and swelling can be considerable. For this reason, and because of the female genital anatomy, the sore may escape notice. In several patients the sore may be high up at the top of the vagina on the neck of the womb (the cervix). It is easy to see how a woman may be unaware of her illness in such a case.

Other sites for the lesion in females are near or on the clitoris or on any other area of adjacent skin of the thighs or lower abdomen, as described in the male.

In both sexes, when the sore has been present for about two to three weeks, the glands in the groins, first on one side, followed a little later by those on the other side, become affected. These again are usually not particularly tender or painful unless the sore is painful. If the patient is thin, the glands are more prominent and he or she is more likely to notice them. If they are not particularly easily seen they may be felt while having a bath.

These glands are part of the body's defence system and their enlargement shows that they have become involved in the disease during their attempt to keep the infection localised. If, in a woman, the sore of primary syphilis is on the cervix, the glands which become infected are deep in the pelvis and the groin glands are not affected. There are thus no outward signs of the infection and unless instruments are used so that the sore can be seen and tests performed on it, the diagnosis of the condition will be missed or delayed. During the delay the infection may spread further in the patient and any sex partner may become affected.

In male homosexuals, the primary sore may be on or near or just inside the anus. It may be quite obvious and discovered by the patient who should then seek advice at a clinic. But the sore may be far from obvious. It may take on the form of a small crack or fissure in the skin. This can easily be unnoticed by the patient or passed off as unimportant. Or it may be misinterpreted. Any lesions at or near the anus are liable to be regarded as "piles". The patient may therefore not seek special advice and may apply various ointments which not only do no good, but may also hinder diagnosis when the lesion is later examined by a doctor.

As with the genitals, the anal canal, the anus and its surrounding skin are protected by the groin lymph glands and swelling of these glands may fortunately lead to the discovery of an unsuspected sore at or near the anus. However, if the sore is in the rectum beyond and higher up than the limits of the anal canal, then the situation is comparable to that in a woman with a sore on the cervix. With a rectal sore, pelvic glands swell and there is thus no outward evidence of disease. It follows that only with the use of instruments enabling the inside of the rectum to be seen, can the sore be discovered and diagnostic tests and treatment be arranged. It can easily be understood that where a man is found to have a syphilitic sore of the penis, then he must tell his sex partner or partners, female or male, that they may well have a hidden infection and should attend for special diagnostic tests without delay.

The problem of the hidden infection in the homosexual is a real one. Whilst undetected and untreated, the disease

86

is progressing in the individual and being passed to contacts. In several centres in Britain, syphilis is more commonly acquired by homosexual contact that by heterosexual. In two London clinics, recent surveys showed that homosexually acquired syphilis formed 70 to 80 per cent of the total new cases seen.

A patient with undiagnosed genital disease may dose himself with antibiotics of one sort or another. They may find some tablets in the bathroom cupboard left over from the treatment of a sore throat or bronchitis, or they may have a cough or heavy cold and can be prescribed tablets by the family doctor. In these and other ways genital disease may be suppressed without any diagnosis having been made. This is bad practice as the treatment may not be the correct one for the disease present and the dose taken may not be enough, so that *the disease may appear to be cured but goes on doing damage and may reappear at a later date. The partially treated patient may also remain infectious or contagious (infection by contact) to others. Similarly, the treatment of sores with various ointments and creams may apparently make them heal yet not cure the underlying disease.*

If the primary sore of syphilis is left untreated, it will heal eventually, taking anything from three to eight weeks, usually about a month. Some time later, say a further month, maybe much longer, the next stage is reached where the attempt of the local lymph glands to control the infection and keep it localised fails, and evidence of spread of disease appears. This is secondary syphilis. Primary and secondary syphilis often overlap and between a quarter and a third of patients showing secondary syphilis may still have an unhealed primary sore.

Secondary syphilis. This is a generalised illness and the organisms have spread to all parts of the body. The patient will probably feel "off colour", generally unwell, perhaps with some fever and headache.

Other features of secondary syphilis are:

(*a*) Skin rash. Most patients show some rash which usually lasts for weeks or months and may come and go. Sometimes it can be fleeting and may pass unnoticed.

The rash is usually a dull red or bronze colour and does not itch. It is equally distributed on each side of the body, back and front. It tends to occur more on the backs of the legs and the front of the arms and may extend on to the face and genitals.

The rash may be just blotches like measles so that it cannot be felt if the fingers are brushed over it, or lumpy so that it can be felt with the eyes shut. These lumps can be quite prominent and behind the scrotum and up around the anus, they may be squashed and rubbed together into bunches like soggy warts. The surface gets rubbed off at times and infected ulcers result. Again, this situation can wrongly be dismissed as "merely piles".

(*b*) With the spread of disease, other groups of lymph glands in various body areas become affected and enlarged. They may be seen and felt commonly in the side, front and back of the neck, in the armpits and less prominently near the elbows. They tend to have the size and feel of small grapes under the skin and occur in over half the patients.

(*c*) Rashes also come in the mouth and throat of about one third of patients. The tops of the spots get rubbed off and ulcers are formed. These may occur on the inside of the lips, on the top of the tongue or under it. If the rash and ulcers affect the tonsils and surroundings there will be sore throats and if the larynx (voice box) is affected, hoarseness may be experienced.

(*d*)   Falling hair is a not uncommon complaint. It may occur from the temples backwards or in patchy areas leaving gaps all over the scalp or there may be a thin general loss noticed in the comb.

(*e*)   Other organs and tissues of the body may occasionally be affected.

Diagnosis and treatment. First, let it be said that all genital sores and anal lumps are not syphilitic in origin. If the penis is trapped in a zip, bleeds a little and then scabs over, the patient has a zip injury, not syphilis. "Cold sores" occur on the penis as they do on the lips and are nothing to do with syphilis. The penis may be bruised or the fraenum get torn at intercourse or it may get sore under the foreskin due to lack of personal cleanliness, or there may be over-enthusiastic use of antiseptics or strong soaps.

There are also other infectious causes of sores not often seen here and more common in other countries. Similarly, there are skin conditions which resemble syphilis but are nothing to do with it. Chief of these are *psoriasis* and *lichen planus.*

On the other hand, if a person has a syphilitic sore or rash this can be diagnosed, treated and cured with ease providing the patient co-operates, and this is not difficult. The first step clinically is for the doctor to suspect the diagnosis from the history of possible infection, the list of contacts, and consideration of the time-relationship of the various events. Supporting evidence is obtained by scraping the sore a little and making it "weep". The fluid is examined down a microscope with special lighting and the *Treponema pallidum* is seen as a moving white spiral.

Similar examination can be made on scrapings of the skin rashes or mouth and throat lesions, or from the anal lumps or rectal sores. If the search is negative, a lymph gland can be punctured with a needle and the fluid examined for *treponemes*. Such a gland-puncture may be necessary if antiseptic ointment has been applied to the primary sore and killed all the surface organisms. In addition to this microscopic help in diagnosis, blood tests may be helpful—although the results are not available for at least four or five days.

Certain special blood tests are at present performed only in what are called Reference Laboratories so the tests are not available for general use. Some blood tests become positive within three weeks of infection; others about four or five weeks after infection; yet another does not react for over two months.

Diagnosis can thus be difficult, and it may be necessary to do more than one set of blood tests before the doctor can be quite sure of his diagnosis. As with primary syphilis, a search for contacts is essential.

Treatment is organised according to the state of the disease. Unless the patient is allergic to Penicillin, the treatment will consist of a number of injections of this drug. The patient calls in each day for a certain number of days according to his type of infection. (The injections are not nearly so bad as imagination suggests and they take only a few seconds!)

If a person is already known to be allergic to Penicillin, another drug can be used for treatment.

If the treatment should fail to cure, and this is highly

unlikely if all the injections are given, the disease can begin to reappear, usually within nine months to two years after treatment. Treated patients are thus followed up for a total period of two years from treatment to make absolutely sure of cure. They need not attend many times during this period of cure-survey, and occasional blood tests and examinations are performed as a check of progress.

At the end of survey, a test is performed at the bottom of the patient's back to make sure the nervous system is normal. Patients may then be discharged or reviewed yearly for a period.

Latent syphilis. If diagnosis and treatment do not occur in the primary or early secondary stages of syphilis, the disease becomes chronic and the symptoms and signs of the secondary stage may come and go for about nine months before the disease becomes quiet and there are no symptoms or signs. This is called latent (meaning hidden) syphilis and these are the types of cases which are sometimes discovered by blood testing on blood donors or pregnant women and on hospital or family practice patients. If the nervous system fluid is also found to be affected, these patients would have latent syphilis of the nervous system. Discovery of such patients leads to accurate assessment, organisation of treatment and careful examination of the sex history followed by a search for contacts.

Because of the diminished numbers of cases, improved diagnosis, treatment and contact tracing and also the frequent use of multiple antibiotic preparations in other diseases, the late stages of syphilis are becoming less and less frequent. Only brief mention will therefore be made of the late signs, particularly as this book is meant for young people who are most unlikely to have the late stages of this disease.

Third stage (tertiary) syphilis. After the onset of latent syphilis the patient remains infectious and such a woman with no outward symptoms or signs may still give birth to a syphilitic baby. Some four years after the original infection, the patient becomes non-infectious but, of course, in the absence of treatment, still has latent un-treated disease. Such a patient may "get away with it" and never have any further trouble, but about a third develop complications later on—anything from five to forty years later—and one-tenth of the total patients will die as a direct result of the disease. In the phase of the disease known as tertiary syphilis, tumours (gummas) appear, commonly in the skin or just under. They tend to ulcerate and form large sores. The patient would almost certainly seek medical help in such a situation and treatment would cure the condition. Of course, if the tumour were in the brain or liver (they can occur anywhere) the patient would be much more seriously ill and treatment might not be so effective.

Fourth stage syphilis (quarternary). In late syphilis (in which gumma is included in some classifications), the heart and blood vessels are mainly attacked. The patient may gradually develop heart failure, or have a sudden heart attack or a stroke. Or the nervous system, which includes the eye, is involved causing partial or com-plete blindness. The patient may have fits or strokes or become insane. Limbs can become paralysed and various body organs function badly. Pain can be severe. Joints may be destroyed and large sores wear away the bottom of the feet even into the bones.

When a patient has such complication, treatment can arrest the infection but not the degenerative changes. The outlook for the patient then depends on how much damage to body tissues has already occurred. Complicated treatments of many types may be required after routine penicillin treatment has been given. Sometimes, surgical operations may be needed and various mechanical devices can be used to assist damaged parts. A man quite badly afflicted may, with patience and retraining, get back to useful work even though he began as a virtual cripple. As stated, such grave complications will never be reached if early diagnosis and treatment are provided.

Untreated syphilis. As a warning, let us now review the trouble which results if a disease as serious as syphilis is NOT treated:

If a woman with untreated infectious syphilis becomes pregnant, the child inside her will be infected. The child's blood circulation is separated from its mother's by a selective filter which prevents the passage of some things but permits others like simple sugars to pass. It also lets *Treponema pallidum* through. Blood passes from the mother's womb through the cord of blood vessels into the child through its navel and after circulating round the baby's body it returns to the mother through the same structures. Two things are clear:

(*a*)   Syphilis organisms in the mother's blood will pass to every tissue in the baby's body.

(*b*)   There is no primary stage and no contact sore. This is a generalised infection at the outset and is equivalent to secondary syphilis in the acquired disease.

The pregnancy may end in miscarriage. Or the baby

may be born at the expected time but is dead at birth, its body swollen and skin bruised and damaged during birth. If the baby is born alive, it will be ill, its cry hoarse and the nose and throat stream with mucus. Sometimes the mouth is ulcerated and blisters may occur on the hands and feet or around the anus and genitals. Some have swollen bones and paralysed limbs.

In yet another type of case, the child may appear normal and gradually develop signs of disease later on in life, when damage to the eyes, nose and teeth will indicate the infection passed to him before he was born. There may be a degree of diminished intelligence if the brain is affected and some deafness. Bones and joints may be involved and tumours (*gummas*) form as in acquired tertiary syphilis. Disease of the nervous system can also develop.

For these children described above in various stages of congenital disease, diagnosis and penicillin treatment are provided. In the new-born, full recovery is anticipated with early treatment. In later stages, antibiotics can stop any infection progressing further. Whatever damage has occurred may be helped by mechanical aids (hearing aids, splints, etc.) and surgical procedures.

The mother of such a child must, of course, be infected and therefore needs treatment. The husband or partner must be traced and anyone who has handled the baby should have blood tests. In a further class of patient with congenital syphilis, there are little or no physical signs of disease and it may only come to light if the blood is tested and found to be positive. This situation is comparable to the patient with latent acquired syphilis.

During pregnancy, tests are essential for the sake of the unborn child and the mother. As infection of the mother may occur after the first set of tests has been shown negative, a second set of tests is indicated late in pregnancy.

Where a mother's blood is found positive and the infection treated during pregnancy, the baby's blood should be tested after it is three months old to make sure that the treatment was successful. During the first three months of life, the baby's blood may still contain some elements of the mother's blood which would give positive tests for syphilis. After this time these elements are eliminated and, providing the mother's treatment was successful, tests on the infant will be negative.

In general, as has been mentioned earlier, patients with sexually transmitted disease or at risk of such infection, should have blood tests both at their first examination and thirteen weeks after the risk to make sure that the tests have not become positive during that time.

Congenital syphilis is rare but still occurs. Some women do not present themselves for blood tests during pregnancy. Not to do so is a serious neglect.

In any system of working, human errors occur—specimens may be wrongly labelled, typists copy incorrectly. These are *technical* false positive reactions. Methods are available to combat such results so that the patients are not wrongly diagnosed. Repeat tests and other check tests are always performed. In other patients, there is no technical error but the patient's blood tests show positive reactions and yet check tests for syphilis performed at the Reference Laboratory show that the patient has, in fact, not got syphilis. There is, however, some underlying cause which may be either unknown or obvious.

Pregnancy is not an uncommon cause or a recent infection such as influenza, or a recent vaccination could be the explanation. Such a blood reaction has nothing to do with syphilis and when the cause resolves, e.g.

pregnancy ends and the woman is delivered of her child, the blood tests gradually become normal again. These patients are said to have an *acute biological* false positive syphilitic blood reaction—false because it has nothing to do with syphilis and acute, meaning it does not last for long.

In a different class are those patients with positive syphilitic blood tests which Reference Laboratory tests show to be nothing to do with syphilis but for which there is usually no obvious cause like pregnancy and which go on and on being positive. These are *chronic* biological false positive reactors, not acute. They may suffer no ill effects although further blood examinations may show other factors which are not in order. In some, there is a history of arthritis or similar rheumatism in a relative or relatives. The patient with the chronic reactions may never suffer any disability but it may be as well if they keep in touch with a doctor so that they can report the development of any rheumatism and treatment can be started at the earliest possible opportunity.

4. TRICHOMONIASIS

This term refers to the symptoms and signs produced by the activity of a small organism called *Trichomonas vaginalis* (T.V. for short). It commonly lives in the vagina, causing no trouble at all and, in some women, the organism seems to live in a sort of carrier state. It is interesting that it is often discovered in the scrapings taken from the cervix when women have a smear test for cancer.

Patients often ask how it gets there in the first place. It has been demonstrated in girls under three weeks old and it is suggested that the baby picks up the organism from an infected mother during the child's passage down the birth-canal when it is being born. The open anatomy of the female child makes it more likely that she will become infected than a boy. An alternative suggestion is that infection is transferred to the baby girl by the hands of an infected mother. Once the organism enters the child's body it apparently usually settles down to a resting state and may only cause symptoms and signs if disturbed. Such a disturbance may occur when the girl reaches puberty, the organism being stimulated by the

TRICHOMONAS VAGINALIS

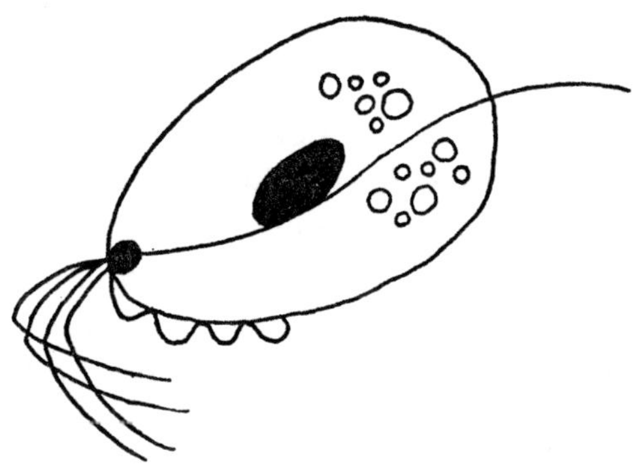

Figure 7

hormone changes which occur at that time and perhaps by commencing menstruation. Or the first sexual intercourse may start symptoms and signs due to Trichomonas. It must be admitted that in such a case, the possibility of a newly acquired infection cannot be denied and some authorities regard T.V. as virtually always sexually introduced.

Certainly, it produces disease much more commonly in the promiscuous and in this group the T.V. is

4—VDE * *

regarded as a cause of sexually transmitted disease. T.V. has been shown to live for a short length of time on wet lavatory seats and wet towels, so chance infection is just a possibility but sex contact or intercourse accounts for most infections. It is also of note that gonorrhoea and Trichomonas commonly occur together in the same patient.

Symptoms and signs. It is in the female that T.V. disease usually produces the most noticeable troubles. True, some women have no symptoms or are able to ignore whatever is present, but in most there is vaginal discharge. This can be slight in amount and accompanied only by vague vaginal discomfort and perhaps a little itching of the skin folds (labia) around the vaginal opening. There may also be a little discomfort when passing urine. In others, the vaginal discharge is increased and some patients may have to change their underclothing several times a day or resort to wearing a sanitary pad, as for menstruation. Where the discharge is pronounced and advice is not sought early, the skin of the labia and groins and thighs can become so sore and chapped that sitting and walking are affected, sexual relations are out of the question and normal life impossible. Uncommonly, infection affects the glands at the urethral opening or in the labia or extends into the pelvis.

At the clinic, specimens of discharge are at once examined by microscope. Trichomonas is usually easily seen, but sometimes, especially where the inflammation of the vagina is severe and the discharge very plentiful, it cannot be found with the microscope, and the diagnosis is only proved by culturing the organism in a laboratory. In such a case, the patient can be treated at her next visit to the clinic when the culture report is known.

Male infection. In men, the symptoms and signs of trichomonal infestation are minimal or absent in most cases. Even in those patients who show some evidence of disease, the trichomonas is often difficult to show under the microscope. However, in the male sex partners of women who have T.V., the organism can sometimes be found, especially if cultures are set up.

T.V. in men is one cause of non-gonococcal urethritis. In other words, it causes inflammation of the urethra in its own right and need not have any connection with gonorrhoea. Symptoms, when present, are sometimes described as a tickling sensation in the urethra. The patient may also complain that he has to go and pass urine more often than normal. There may be no visible discharge or there may be a little mucoid stickiness at the urethral opening. In others, there is a mattery discharge, as in N.S.U.

At the clinic, tests must be made on urethral discharge, as in the female. A swab specimen is also taken and sent to the laboratory so that check tests and cultures may show the organism even if it is not found in the clinic. In those men who have no discharge but complain of vague dysuria, or are anyway known to have been in sex contact with a woman who has T.V., a slide sample is taken by gently scraping the urethra with a platinum wire bent into a tiny loop (by the way, this is not nearly as unpleasant as it sounds and is an essential part of proper medical care).

Spread of infection is not common in either sex but has been reported. Similar to the complications of non-specific genital infection, spread of T.V. in women may cause pelvic infection, and similarly, as in men with N.S.U., may cause epididymitis, prostatitis or other genital or pelvic complications.

Treatment. This is simple in either sex: a course of tablets is given, one tablet to be taken three times daily for a week, or two can be taken only twice a day, morning and night, and this may offer advantages to patients who are forgetful about taking a tablet to work to take at midday. Patients should not have intercourse until they are cured.

If there is a regular sex partner, they should receive a contact slip and be seen at the clinic, and, if necessary, treated at the same time as their partner. If the T.V. is not found, they can be offered the treatment as a precaution. If the partners cannot be treated at the same time, they should not have sexual intercourse until treatment has in fact been completed for both of them, otherwise the T.V. will repeatedly pass from the untreated to the treated partner and the disease will begin all over again. The same is true, of course, for gonorrhoea and syphilis. Even if the original patient has not got a regular sex partner, a contact slip is provided for each of any recent contacts so that they can be examined and any necessary treatment given. Only in this way can the spread of disease be controlled.

5. THRUSH

Infection of the genital and urinary passages with Thrush fungus is a common cause of illness and can be sexually transmitted. The fungus infection is also known as Moniliasis or Candidosis.

The Thrush fungus grows well in sugary surroundings and if a patient has Thrush, the urine is especially tested for sugar, perhaps on repeated occasions. An enquiry will be made about sugar diabetes in the patient's relatives, as diabetes runs in families. However, Thrush occurs as a genital or urinary infection in the absence of sugar and may be the cause of much discomfort in either sex.

Symptoms and signs. In the female, Thrush is a common cause of vaginal irritation and discharge. The inflammation may be mild, moderate or so severe as to cause pain and bleeding. As the infected discharge overflows on to the surrounding skin of the labia, the groins,

THRUSH   FUNGUS

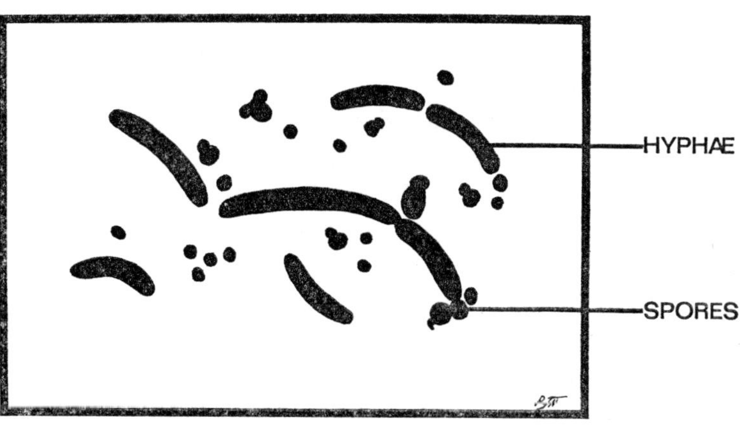

Figure 8

thighs and lower abdomen all these areas may become inflamed, especially in women who are overweight. Where discharge is visible at the vaginal entrance and surrounding area, the patient may notice white flecks and blobs, rather like the soft curd which separates from the liquid in sour milk. Itching can be intense. As itchy skin is worse when one is warm, the condition is often worse in bed and the patient may get little sleep. This lowers her general resistance and increases irritability still further and she can get into a very harassed state, both mentally and physically.

To add to the difficulties, the passage of urine through such inflamed surroundings inevitably results in some degree of stinging. The rectum may also become infected, indeed the bowel may be the source of the original infection, especially if the patient has been taking certain types of tablets. In rectal and anal infections, anal itching can be severe. The vagina is very red and sore with flecks of discharge. All the area of skin affected is red, itchy and sore. It may become cracked and bleeding. Uncontrolled scratching leads to more damage and possibly secondary skin infection.

In the male, as with T.V., Thrush may cause non-gonococcal urethritis and give rise to a variable degree of discomfort and urethral discharge.

Commonly though, and especially in men who have not been circumcised and still have a foreskin covering the glans penis, the infection occurs under the foreskin rather than in the urethra. The fungus causes considerable discomfort, with itching under the foreskin. There is often some discharge of watery, sticky matter and quite severe inflammation, so that the surface of the glans, and the inside of the foreskin become bright red, shiny, sore and may bleed.

This condition is called balanitis and is often severe in people with sugar diabetes. Many diabetics develop their sugar diabetes very slowly and the bright red inflammation due to Thrush growing in the sugary urine which seeps under the foreskin may be the first indication of their underlying disease.

Especially in elderly and overweight men, the infection can spread over the skin of the penis and scrotum into the groins and pubic region.

Treatment. Where the appearance fits the above description, the diagnosis is suspected from the clinical signs and the complaint of severe itch. Swab samples, especially from the vagina in women and under the foreskin in men, can be taken as well as examining male urethral discharge. Additionally, specimens from these body areas are sent for laboratory testing, and rectal specimens are indicated if the skin round the anus is very itchy and inflamed. Rectal infection may be more likely if the patient has had certain antibiotics by mouth. Such may be the case where a man has been treated for N.S.U.

Through the microscope the Thrush fungus appears as blue threads and blue, oval spores, usually described as flask-shaped. Where the infection seems limited to a surface structure, such as under the foreskin or inside the vagina, local treatment with creams may be sufficient to deal with the situation.

Treatment in women with vaginal infection may be strengthened by the use of pessaries—special tablets made to be pushed high up into the vagina. If there is deeper infection, such as a Thrush urethritis or infection of the rectum, tablets can be taken by mouth to kill the fungus.

As with other diseases affecting the sex-organs and nearby areas, arrangements are made to examine and treat sex-partners. The urine of all new patients is tested for sugar, perhaps on repeated occasions.

In addition to its association with diabetes, Thrush can also be connected with pregnancy, injury, thyroid disease and malnutrition. It can occur in couples where the woman is taking the contraceptive pill. Its relation to antibiotics treatments has been mentioned and it can also be related to various cancers, including blood cancers. And it occurs as a sex-connected disease in otherwise normal individuals. It is thus obvious that each case needs assessment on its own merits.

6. ABNORMAL DISCHARGES

The causes of urethral discharge in men have been quite fully discussed in the sections of this book describing gonorrhoea, non-gonococcal urethritis and N.S.U. Rectal emissions in gonorrhoea and syphilis have been mentioned.

In women, gonorrhoea and T.V. account for most abnormal vaginal discharges. Thrush, as dealt with on page 101, and non-specific cervicitis is commonly associated with varying amounts of vaginal discharge. Another frequent source of discharge is objects placed in the vagina for one reason or another—contraception, sanitation, etc. The coil, loop or diaphragm may all cause discharge. Ring pessaries inserted for prolapse of the uterus (fallen womb) are also often to blame. Tampons and other neglected sanitary wear may cause profuse foul-smelling discharge.

Some women douche the vagina for sanitary and/or contraceptive reasons. Vaginal discharge and discomfort may result. This is especially so if strong soaps or anti-septic solutions are used and it is often the perfume in soap which causes the inflammation. The same applies to some of the recently marketed aerosol "deodorants" which both women and men are currently using to spray the genital region! Quite severe vaginal irritation and discharge may result in women and marked skin irritation in both sexes. Contraceptive creams can have similar results.

Hormones are natural chemicals which govern the proper function of the body and alteration in their balanced state can cause vaginal discharge. Such alteration occurs during menstruation, and many young women see a regular moderate increase in discharge before a period. Pregnancy also alters the hormone balance and again some vaginal discharge is common. Psychological trouble such as worry and anxiety can also be a cause.

As stated earlier, some vaginal discharge may be a normal feature of some women's lives. If it is excessive, if it causes discomfort, if it soils clothing and makes changes of underwear necessary, or if it alters from its normal pattern, then you should see a doctor.

6

Other Sexually Transmitted Diseases

I. WARTS

THE appearance of warts on the hands is familiar enough, usually on the fingers and backs of the hands. Warts are lumps of various sizes with a scaly, hard, often dirty surface which, on close inspection is seen to be made up of separate closely packed parts. In moist areas warts are softer and in rubbing together may be damaged and infected.

Warts affecting the genital areas may be (*a*) rough and lumpy, (*b*) smooth and flat, and (*c*) smooth and dome-shaped.

(*a*)   These are the usual type of wart known to most people in the form just described. In men, they tend to occur on the shaft of the penis, on the foreskin, or under it. In women, they tend to occur at the vaginal entrance or just inside or on the folds of skin (labia) surrounding. Or they may be high up on the cervix, out of sight. In both sexes they may surround the anus. In a woman this may be because wart infection gets swept backwards to the anus from the vaginal region when she lies on her back.

Warts are an infectious condition caused by a

WARTS

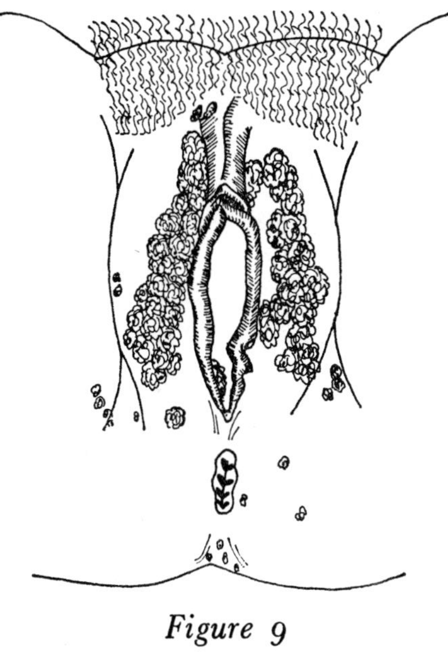

Figure 9

virus. Genital warts are presumed to be associated with sexual intercourse probably in 90 per cent of cases. There is doubt whether they can be transmitted from hand to genitals during sex-play. Anal and rectal warts are probably associated with anal intercourse in women or men. Of partners admitting such intercourse, not many have genital warts so the mechanism of anal infection needs further explanation. Untreated, warts can heal themselves in weeks or months. Often they become chronic, grow larger and spread. They may become very large and troublesome. In a man, the whole foreskin may be involved, inside or outside or both, so that the foreskin cannot be pulled back. In a woman, they can form a large pad like a small cauliflower which obscures the vaginal entrance and surroundings. In both cases there may be bleeding and secondary bacterial infection.

Treatment involves the application of a chemical solution regularly (say two or three times weekly) to the genital and anal warts. Healing may take place in two or three weeks or longer.

Hand warts need freeze treatment and the patient will have to attend a skin clinic, where the expensive freeze treatment is available once or twice a week at special wart clinics.

In both sexes, electrical heat treatment may be needed if the genital warts do not respond to chemical measures. Surgical operation, including circumcision (cutting off most of the foreskin) is sometimes performed on the male.

Warts around the vagina are fairly common in pregnancy. If these do not respond to chemical treatment, they can be ignored as they never seem to affect the childbirth or the baby itself and will probably clear up after baby is born.

(b) *Flat* warts on the genitals are uncommon, usually affect the surface of the shaft or glans of penis in men and heal spontaneously or with simple chemical treatment. Several may be found lying in a straight line and may occur in scratch marks or other minor injuries.

(c) This lesion, caused by a virus, may be regarded as a type of wart. It often occurs on people's bodies and seems commonly to be caught at swimming baths, either in the water or from towels or swimming costumes. Sometimes it occurs solely on the genitals, in which case it may be sexually transmitted. Some experts think the infecting virus may be carried by pubic lice. If it spreads, a patient may get hundreds of the tiny dome-shaped lesions with a little pit on the top of each: the condition is known as Molluscum Contagiosum.

Treatment is usually simple by chemical or freeze methods and should involve the sex partner if necessary. It must be repeated despite earlier coverage in this book; secondary syphilis in the ano-genital area can look very like warts.

2. SCABIES

This catching, itching disease (it is known as the "itch") is caused by a tiny animal or mite—a parasite in fact—living just inside the human skin. Its life cycle is interesting: the male fertilises a female and then dies. The female burrows around in the skin surface laying about four eggs a day for eight weeks—then she too dies. The eggs hatch and small new animals or nymphs grow up. They lose their skin once or twice and become males or females. Then the process begins again.

Infection occurs by adult acarus males and females, or fertilised females alone or even nymphs, passing from one person to another. Some closeness for a certain length of time is thus required, and the warmth of bed makes transfer easier as the acarus dies without human body heat. Thus the disease is very often regarded as sexually transmitted.

The female acarus selects the body areas on which to lay its eggs. These areas are on the genitals, buttocks, wrists, ankles, the spaces between the fingers and toes and near the armpits. Young children also get lesions on

ACARUS OF SCABIES

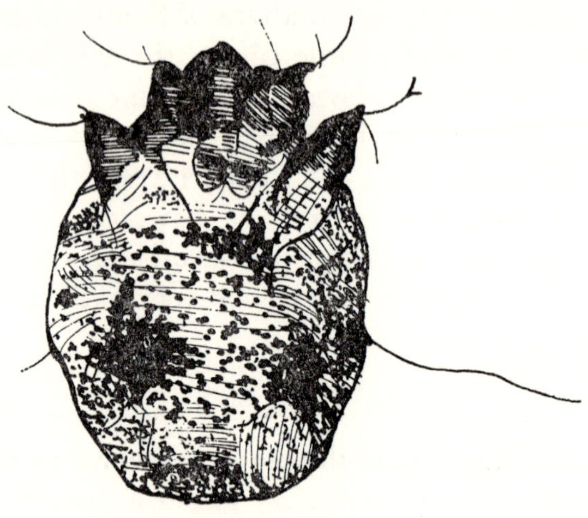

Figure 10

the face, palms and soles. Itchy lumps form in the infected areas and are often specially pronounced on the genitals and buttocks. The minute tracks made by the mite burrowing in the skin may be seen if scratching has not destroyed them. Later, after a few weeks, the patient may become sensitised to the invading bug and a more generalised skin eruption occurs.

Diagnosis is made by the typical appearance of the rash and burrows and is supported by a history of contact with the disease. The acarus can be picked out of the skin with a pin and some doctors like to make certain of the diagnosis by this method.

Treatment involves covering the skin from the neck to the toe ends with a lotion provided by the clinic. It is best if the lotion is put on after a hot bath as the hot water softens the skin and the lotion penetrates more effectively. This treatment is usually repeated the following day, after which all the clothes the patient has been wearing are hung on a hook for two days and the clothes of his bed thrown back and the bed left open from the time he leaves it in the morning until he goes to bed that night. This lets all clothing cool down so no acarus could survive. It is not necessary to go to the expense of boiling or cleaning everything.

All sex contacts should be seen and treated even if nothing is found, as the infection is very easily caught and contacts will often develop the disease later even if they show nothing when first examined. Ideally, all the members of a household or flat should be treated if one member is affected.

It should be understood that if any area of the skin is left untreated, it is likely that the treatment will fail and the itch and rash will return.

3. PUBIC LICE

"Crabs", to use the popular name, is an infestation of the human body with the pubic louse (*Phthirus pubis*). These, like the acarus of scabies, soon die without human body heat and nourishment (they feed on skin and blood). They mainly occur attached to the base of the hairs around the genital and anal regions but they can be found on the abdomen and chest in hairy people. They may also be found in the armpits, on the eyebrows and eyelashes and occasionally in men attached to the hair on the tops of the fingers and toes.

Pubic lice occurring outside the genital region may have spread by wandering or by transfer on the fingers. Transfer from person to person as the distribution indicates, is always (or almost always) sexual.

If, as we did previously with the acarus, we look at the life-cycle of the parasite it helps considerably in understanding the infestation of the human body.

Male and female "crabs" have sexual intercourse and two days later the female starts to lay three or four fertilised eggs a day for a week. These eggs are the "nits" which are just visible to the naked eye, each attached to

THE CRAB LOUSE

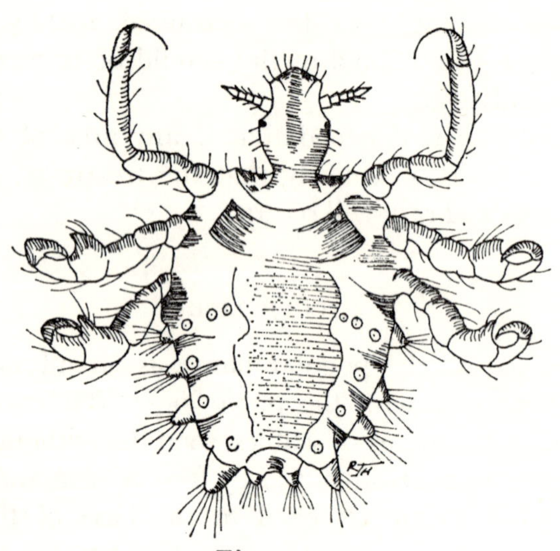

Figure 11

a single pubic hair about an inch up from the skin. These "nits" hatch in a week and babies (or larvae) grow during the next fortnight into adults and the process then repeats itself. Transfer of larvae and adult forms from person to person occurs during body contact or in a shared bed.

It usually happens that a patient will be infected for about a month before symptoms and signs are noted.

Symptoms and signs. About half the infected people seeking treatment complain either of itch or seeing "insects", or both complaints. Adult crab lice are about the width of an average matchstick and thus fairly easily seen when roving free in the pubic hair. When half buried in the skin at the base of a hair during feeding, they are less easily detected. Being a brownish colour they tend to look like freckles and some patients do come to the doctor complaining that they have "spots" of recent origin. Perhaps two out of ten patients found with crabs have no symptoms or, at least, make no complaint—this is surprising as many others say that the itch is "maddening".

The patient with "crabs" may complain of an entirely different sex disease and it is common to find pubic lice associated with, say, gonorrhoea. Indeed it is not really uncommon to find multiple disease in the same patient. A woman may attend clinic complaining of vaginal discharge and be found to have gonorrhoea, T.V. and scabies. A man may complain of urethral discharge and is found to have gonorrhoea, scabies, crabs and genital warts.

Treatment. Lotion is provided. It is usually **D.D.T.** or a similar poison. It should be applied liberally and rubbed into the hairs from the level of the navel to the knees, especially in the pubic area and all over and around the genitals and between the buttocks. It should be applied in both armpits and rubbed on to the chest and upper abdomen in hairy individuals. Nits in other sites mentioned may require treatment. The lotion should be left in place for at least two days, preferably three. If washing occurs during that time, as in miners who must shower, the lotion must be re-applied. For each day of treatment, the bed-clothes should be thrown right back and the bed left open for the day. Any "crabs" seen on the under sheets may be picked off with the fingers and dropped down the sink or out of the window.

At the end of the treatment period, the lotion is washed off as mentioned previously, and the discarded clothes hung away for at least two days. Boiling and cleaning are not necessary. Underwear is washed normally. Some brown speckling of the inside of the pants may be difficult to wash away. This does not matter: it is not infectious and is only staining caused during the infection. The pants need not be thrown away and the stains will fade.

All sex-partners should be seen: contact slips will be provided. Non-sexual bed-partners should also be invited to attend clinic. One last point: the pubic and genital hair should not be shaved because:

(1)   It probably will not remove all the lice and eggs, so it is not effective.
(2)   Serious cuts can occur. In any case, multiple scratch injuries occur during shaving and when treatment is applied it enters the injured areas and can be very pain-ful.
(3)   It does not make treatment more effective.
(4)   In removing many of the invaders it makes diagnosis more difficult.
(5)   The period during which the hairs are re-growing can be highly uncomfortable.

4. "COLD" SORES

It is not generally appreciated that "cold sores" (*Herpes Simplex*) can affect the genital organs and their surround-ings as well as occurring around the mouth. There are two viruses, Type I and Type II. Type I causes the usual type of cold sore on the lips. It is thought to be acquired in early life and the patient then becomes a carrier, the virus lying in a resting state in various areas such as the mouth, eyes and nose. During a time of upset, such as a heavy "cold" in the head, menstruation, and even in response to strong sunlight, the virus becomes reactivated and produces symptoms and signs. Type II virus inhabits the genitals and is responsible for sexually transmitted "cold-sores" of the sex-organs: it can occasionally affect the mouth also.

In the male, the condition usually affects the penis glans and foreskin; in the female the vaginal entrance and surroundings.

Symptoms and signs. Both men and women usually feel a prickly sensation in the affected area, then small blisters form. These soon burst, especially in areas where they are subjected to pressure and friction, as under the foreskin. They may thus be so short-lived that the patient does not notice them. Having burst, shallow rounded ulcers are left, and the groin glands of one or both sides draining the area become enlarged. Several of the small ulcers may grow together to form a larger open sore. Secondary bacterial infection leads to a yellow crust forming on the top of the sore which now becomes quite painful and the groin glands become similarly painful and tender.

To the doctor, the history and clinical appearance are of the greatest help. Swabs from the sore can be sent to the laboratory for identification of the virus.

Treatment. There is no specific treatment. Washing with soap and water and a weak salt solution will usually help healing in about a week. Secondary bacterial infection may need a little antibiotic cream. Recurrent attacks occur just as "cold" sores tend to recur around the lips in some people. Nothing is known which prevents such recurrences.

The physician is however, wary of genital sores and scrape examinations can be made to exclude the presence of syphilis.

OTHER GENITAL SORES

Genital sores due to particular specified organisms are now rarities.

Chancroid or soft sore is caused by a bacterium. The sufferer (male usually) gets a penile sore and the groin glands swell. The glands may fester and discharge through the skin of the groin. Much damage to the penis can occur. Effective treatment is available. The disease is uncommon here and occurs mainly in the East and in South America.

L.G.V. (*Lymphogranuloma venereum*) is also uncommon here. A virus disease, it has a fleeting primary sore which may be missed. Groin swelling and considerable pelvic disorder may follow. There may be later great swelling of the genitals. Negroid and related races are usually involved.

Granuloma inguinale is a parasitic disease rarer still and of low infectivity. A spreading sore develops on the genitals or nearby. It is probably a sexually transmitted disease, but this is only presumed from the site of infection.

Traumatic. The penis may suffer injury in various ways. Probably commonest is the fraenular tear. Usually during intercourse the fraenum is ripped across due to overstretching. An ulcer results: it often gets secondarily infected and can be very painful indeed. It may be accompanied by some swelling in the region.

Another common cause of penile sore is zip-fastener injury. This often results in a scab, or there may be one or two such scars in line. They usually heal without difficulty but are often very sore for a time, especially if they become infected. This type of injury is commonly acquired just after a man has passed urine. It would not occur if the man wore underpants and the penis was replaced inside the underwear before the zip was re-fastened. It is commoner after taking alcohol and in such circumstances, the man may not realise the injury has occurred. In both these conditions regular gentle washing will lead to improvement and a little antibiotic cream may help healing and diminish soreness.

Balanitis. Mention has been made of this in the discussion on Thrush. Inflammation under the foreskin may also occur if regular washing is not performed. The operation of circumcision, usually performed in childhood when the foreskin is judged to be too tight, removes most of the foreskin and leaves most of the glans of the penis open to the air. This means that any secretions produced by the special skin glands in this area do not accumulate. In uncircumcised men, white secretion tends to collect under the foreskin, especially in the groove at the base of the glans.

This white secretion (smegma) can act as an irritant, especially if it becomes bacterially infected. Several organisms found about the human body can be responsible. Apart from bacteria, some spirochaetes (not the *Treponema pallidum* of syphilis) may be the cause of the trouble and T.V. may also contribute to the inflammation. Various chemicals may cause balanitis. It is not uncommonly due to antiseptic lotions, creams and soaps. Even the perfume in some soaps can produce similar effects. Perfumes and antiseptics in some "deodorant" sprays are a cause and even the volatile liquid base of such toilet preparations can act as sufficient irritant in some susceptible males.

Men should regularly pull the foreskin right back and wash the end of the penis clean. All soap should be washed away or this may also cause inflammation as indicated above. The penis should be dried gently before pulling the foreskin down again into its normal position.

It is important to replace the foreskin to the down position (this also applies after sexual intercourse) as it may become very swollen and painful, even ulcerated, if left in the drawn-back position. A surgical opinion can be sought if the foreskin is so tight that it cannot be pulled back (*phimosis*).

7

Skin Conditions

A variety of skin conditions must be considered in such a book as this. Indeed, many of these patients go to special Treatment Clinics because the genital region is affected or, in the case of widespread rashes without genital lesions, people who have put themselves at risk and are worried about sexually transmitted diseases.

Despite much current ignorance of sexual disorders, many patients know that "V.D. and skin diseases are connected". It is true, of course, that different types of skin rash may be associated with syphilis and it is thus not surprising that patients bring skin lesions for opinion. Family doctors also refer skin conditions, especially where the sexual history is suspicious.

Of the skin rashes, the commonest appearing are:

Psoriasis: Red areas with dry greyish white scales. Various sizes from small dots to large map-like areas. They tend to bleed if the scales are scratched off. Common over the bends of joints, body and limbs, in the scalp and can affect nails. Sometimes affects the groins and can appear on the genitals alone. Often occurs in relatives.

Lichen planus: Small (pin-head) spots like purplish flat warts with fine silvery lines running over them. Or can appear as pinkish-purple rings raised above the skin surface. If many spots fuse together purple patches form on the skin. It can appear widespread or in small localised areas. White areas inside the mouth may be somewhat painful. It can occur on the penis, sometimes as the sole lesion.

Seborrhoeic dermatitis: Red, sometimes rather greasy skin patches in people with "oily skins" and a tendency to head scurf (dandruff). Common in skin-contact areas including armpits, between buttocks and in the groins. Can occur in pubic area and affect the genitals.

Eczema: Childhood eczema can persist to adult life and the groins and genitals may well be affected. Eczematous reactions on the genitals (pink scaling sometimes with blistering, weeping and itch) may result from contact with various substances including rubber sheath contraceptives and various contraceptive or "deodorant" chemicals.

"Athlete's foot": Soggy cracking skin between and under the toes especially attacks those who use communal bathing facilities with cracked tile or concrete floors (e.g. pithead baths and swimming bath showers) where the fungus causing the disease lives. The same fungus can cause large red scaling areas in one or both groins, often spreading on to the thighs rather than on to the scrotum.

Pityriasis rosea: Reddish oval areas with fine ring of scales. Occurring mainly on the trunk it can be concentrated at skin folds, e.g. in the groins, although the genitals are little if at all affected.

Pityriasis versicolor: Small or widespread areas of tan coloured pigmentation with fine scaling especially over the upper trunk. Caused by a fungus, it causes depigmentation in Negroes so the colour-scheme is reversed and the affected areas are paler than the normal skin. The genital area escapes.

Shingles: This may occur in adults in contact with children with chicken-pox (same virus) or there may be no such contact history. Angry blisters with red surrounds get infected and often progress to matter-filled spots. Affects the face and eye or chest or abdomen or limb. Can affect the genitals, sometimes only in this site. Pain can be severe.

Accidental vaccination: Those in contact with children recently vaccinated against smallpox should beware transferring vaccination material from the baby's arm to their genitals. Troublesome pock-marks may result, at first pus-filled spots, later sores with black craters.

Most of these conditions can be cured: all can be helped. Some clinics carry a fairly full stock of treatments. In other clinics it is the policy to exclude sexually related disease and then advise the patient to attend his family doctor or be referred to a skin-disease clinic.

Patients do not always realise that since the formation of the Health Service in 1948, sexually transmitted diseases and skin diseases are dealt with in separate clinics, although certainly these fields of medicine overlap. But you can rest assured that whatever you have wrong, when you visit a clinic the best attempt will be made to manage the condition there or to advise you where best to attend in future.

Nothing to worry about. Many skin markings have nothing to do with disease. They have usually been present all the patient's life and are only discovered during a bout of self-examination, usually following some casual sexual escapade which (when the heat of the moment has passed) becomes a matter for regret and anxiety.

There are four main pit-falls:

(1)   There is a ring of multiple white or pink dots, all much the same size, clustered around the lower border of the glans where it dips into the groove (or sulcus) below. In some men they are prominent enough to appear as short stalks, again all lying together approximately the same size. These are normal glands. All men have them. No disease.

(2)   The skin of the shaft of the penis and the foreskin and the skin of the scrotum contains small (size of two pin heads) white glands. These are usually seen best when the skin is put slightly on the stretch. The same type of structure and appearance may be seen in the folds (labia) around the vaginal opening in women. Again, these are normal structures, common to all. No disease.

(3)   The genitals and surrounding skin are quite common sites for moles—brown or bluish markings that are usually birth marks or appear soon after. These are, of course, nothing to do with infection of any sort, let alone sexually transmitted infection.

(4)   The scrotum in men is sometimes dotted with red spots. These are inherited spots composed of blood-vessels. Again, no disease.

Three further sources of needless anxiety may be set down here:

(*a*)   The genital area in both sexes is commonly of darker colour than the rest of the body. This is normal.

(*b*)   The erect penis is noted to have prominent veins on its surface. A penis becomes erect due to increased blood flow. Therefore the veins must be full of blood and bulging. Normal.

(*c*) The genitals, in men and women, have a different smell characteristic of the sex. This is normal and can play a part in sexual arousal. Daily local washing may be indicated to prevent offence.

8

Girls at Risk

AT PRESENT, well over 50,000 new cases of gonorrhoea are being recorded every year and the trend is upwards.

The 1968 figure was 7.1 per cent more than 1967
The 1969 figure was 13.9 per cent more than 1968
The 1970 figure was 4.4 per cent more than 1969

One in every six patients with gonorrhoea is under twenty years old. In the patients under twenty, there are so many girls and young women that they amount to one-third of all new female patients with gonorrhoea.

	NEW INFECTIONS WITH GONORRHOEA					
	Under 16 years			Over 16 under 20 years		
	Male	*Female*	*Total*	*Male*	*Female*	*Total*
1968	69	215	284	2845	3054	5899
1969	72	331	403	3486	3792	7278
1970	80	395	475	4106	5104	9210

These figures reflect the great increase in sexual activity in the young and in girls in particular, especially those under sixteen. It had commonly been the case in past years for new male patients attending clinics to out-number females by as much as 4 to 1. In many clinics, these figures are tending to equalise and in some the number of new female patients actually exceeds the new males.

Many such girls come from disturbed family backgrounds, and, for the rest, many feel discontented with their lives. Others attempt to opt out of family life as much as possible. Nowadays, even in apparently good and stable homes, the young of both sexes often feel little contact with their parents. Guidance from parents is in many instances lacking.

Not knowing quite what they are seeking, many young girls run away from home. Others who are old enough, or look it, join the pub-sets and club-sets. Young people of both sexes face a world in which diminished parental control combines with the influences of what is called "the permissive society". Films, television, literature and radio all have an increased content of sexual activity which varies from objective reporting to lurid distortion.

Such an atmosphere sets the stage for promiscuity, and a higher incidence of gonorrhoea is one result. Other factors which tend to keep the infection rate high can also be readily understood. For instance, as this book has already explained to you, many girls with early infections have no symptoms or signs. If they run away from home and move from place to place having casual intercourse they can pass the disease on to several men before they have any hint of infection. The fact that they are moving about the country makes them difficult to trace.

The same can be said about rectally infected male homosexuals and, to a less extent, those symptomless men with urethral infection. Women taking the contraceptive pill and those fitted with a coil or loop (intra-uterine device) may also exhibit more sexual freedom than they would otherwise. To a less extent, this applies also to pregnant women.

On the medical side, a further factor in today's high incidence of gonorrhoea is growing resistance of the causative organism to Penicillin. The gonococcus is gradually adapting itself to withstand this drug. Resistance to some other treatments has also developed. This means that the infection may not respond at all to the treatment provided, or it may appear to respond initially and then the discharge returns. During the time of apparent cure it is not uncommon for a patient to resume sexual intercourse either with a regular partner or on a casual basis. This spreads the disease and spreads drug-resistant organisms also.

With the increase in sexual activity in all sections of society, the part played by the female prostitute in the spread of gonorrhoea is diminishing; indeed in one group of men with gonorrhoea the source of the infection came from prostitutes in only 12 per cent. At the present time, however, they still provide considerable risk.

It has to be admitted that in the sphere of non-specific urethritis and non-specific genital infection the situation remains unsatisfactory. Although a diagnosis may be reached in the male and treatment provided, the condition—as I have said earlier—is still not properly understood. The cause is not established, and the condition is difficult to define and diagnose in women.

Syphilis has been reviewed. Judged purely on numbers this may seem an inconsiderable, even unimportant, infection compared with gonorrhoea and N.S.U. The fact that its late complications are less and less seen also tends to remove this disease from public consciousness. Indeed, many young patients seen at clinic at the present time have never heard of the disease. It must be taught and remembered that this sexually transmitted disease still exists.

Probably the greatest risk of infection lie in the prostitute and in homosexuals. It is commonest in promiscuous individuals, usually in an older age group.

9

The Future

THE control of gonorrhoea must depend to a large extent on early diagnosis and treatment and on successful contact tracing.

Where patients with obvious clinical symptoms and signs present themselves for examination, management of the illness is usually rapidly achieved. Difficulty arises where the patient feels well or is reluctant to be examined.

A simple diagnostic test which did not involve genital examination would obviously be of great assistance in such cases. A blood test, as is used for screening patients for syphilis, would be suitable. Research along these lines has been made but so far has proved unproductive.

On the tracing of contacts the public, young people in particular, should realise what a powerful force they could exert to bring about a large measure of control of this disease.

It is usually the infected male who first presents at clinic. Many of these young men, having been treated, realise that the girl from whom they acquired their infection is ill and does not know it. Although they may feel resentful at first, often they realise that they have a public duty to try and bring the girl for treatment. Where the infecting female is not properly known, the man may be able to describe where she lives (or which pub or cafe she frequents). A special form is available and if properly completed, provides good descriptive information about the infected person.

In this search for the sexual partner, the assistance of a special nurse or health visitor is most valuable and in addition more major clinics are being provided with Welfare Officers to share the work-load. It is taxing, painstaking work but so obviously worthwhile and it is hoped that more nurses will enter this important field.

It must be admitted, however, that where the young girl is "on the run", contact tracing becomes virtually impossible. The casual heterosexual or homosexual pick-up of short-time nature in the busy city is also similarly difficult to trace.

The fact that babies are still developing gonorrhoea of the eyes shortly after being born provides yet another indication of undetected infection in women. The infected women whose babies get the eye infection have often had no proper supervision of their pregnancy (ante-natal care). It is the duty of every pregnant woman to accept the medical care provided for her and her unborn child. She should attend her family doctor who can refer her to an ante-natal clinic. Here, any abnormal discharge should be examined. It is not current practice to test pregnant mothers for sexually transmitted diseases other than syphilis. Time and facilities are not so organised.

It may in future be thought wise to arrange such tests as a routine part of ante-natal care, especially with increasing promiscuity, unmarried pregnant women and the increasing number of requests for abortions. (The development of a diagnostic blood test or similar simple screening test for gonorrhoea as mentioned earlier should be ideal for such circumstances.)

Drug resistance. The problem of drug-resistant

5—VDE

organisms is constantly under survey. This is essential to the proper control of gonorrhoea as, in some parts of the world, outbreaks of the disease are prevelant in which 60 per cent or more of the infections are due to organisms which show some resistance to penicillin treatment. (This penicillin resistance fortunately does not occur in syphilis.)

Penicillin treatment in sexually transmitted diseases is given by injection into muscle, and there are three good reasons for this:

(1)   The doctor knows the exact dose provided and that all that dose has gone inside the patient;
(2)   tablets may upset the patient's stomach and may in part be passed out with the motion when he moves his bowel; and
(3)   tablets may be lost, given away, thrown away or forgotten.

In (2) and (3) above the dosage is not known and the infection may only be partially treated. For these reasons what is required for the future, both for the Penicillin-resistant gonococcus and for use in patients who cannot have Penicillin because they are allergic to it, is another injectable drug. This drug will have to kill the gonococcus without harming the patient and be cheap enough for the Health Service to be able to stand the cost. Work goes on in this direction.

More research is needed in N.S.U., not particularly into treatment but to find the cause. Some work has been done and there are indications that many cases are due to a virus. It is hoped further study will clarify the position. Only when the cause, or causes, are properly known, can work be organised to produce a specific cure, possibly diminishing or abolishing the recurrent attacks which prove so troublesome in many men. More research into a better technique for studying and isolating T.V. in men might be helpful.

Yet another field in which research might provide control of the sexually transmitted diseases is that of immunology. Indications show that it might be possible to produce a vaccine so that people could be immunised against these infections. The work is hardly begun.

It should be said also that even if a vaccine were produced its administration to the public would create certain social and ethical problems—who should receive it, at what age? Social attitudes are changing so fast that further speculation is pointless.

In another field, the study of behavioural sciences may be employed to demonstrate "at-risk" groups for special consideration and protection.

On a practical level what we can see is the amount of work which has to be done to try and control these diseases. In the less important but often troublesome conditions, warts could provide a worthwhile study. Their behaviour is very imperfectly understood.

Although warts are caused by a virus, the infection does not seem to be followed by any lasting immunity and patients get recurrent attacks. It is also unexplained why they can heal in one area of the body whilst appearing in another, as if any immunity associated with them were a purely local feature. It is also unexplained why they heal rapidly with little treatment in some patients while persisting for months or years in others, despite repeated and prolonged treatment.

Adequate attack upon the present problem of the sexually transmitted diseases will probably depend upon two main factors—money and recruitment of more workers in the field at all levels—nurses, technicians, clinical doctors and laboratory specialists.

V.D. Explained

Ultimate control of the sexually transmitted diseases may lie in change in public attitude. Members of a community can only reach rational decisions if they are well informed. Whilst some local authorities in this country have appointed full-time Health Education Officers, some of whom promote very active programmes in their localities, this whole subject must be admitted to be in its infancy.

The Health Education Council has as its task the promotion and organisation of a comprehensive scheme so that young people are well informed on basic anatomy and human body function. Sex education forms only a part of a major study which should include instruction and explanation about acceptable community living as seen in the context of our society.

Some appropriate headings for a programme of Health Education and Community Living may be found in the following:

Mental Health and body fitness
Community Life
The individual in society: respect for other people
Your job and other people's: recreations
Growing up
Puberty: menstruation: male puberty
Sexual attraction: love
Choosing a partner
Sexual function: use and abuse
Marriage: its benefits and responsibilities
   Home-making
   Birth control
   Sex techniques
   Sexually transmitted diseases
   Pregnancy

Childbirth
Abortion
Bringing up children

Whilst my list may not be comprehensive, I hope it gives an idea of the scope involved in a drive towards a successful society involving parents, teachers, youth leaders and many others who seek to help young people with problems to face in a world of increasing pace and complexity.

It is a problem of today's society that sexual drive and power appear in young people who have not the worldly capacity to deal with it. They have no jobs, either being still at school or as yet without employment, or—even if they are at work—earning little money. Such young people can thus not afford to settle together, set up house or flat, buy furniture, clothing, kitchen goods or food. They are not in a position to care for any children.

This is not a new problem, but is arriving earlier now that boys and girls are reaching physical maturity up to two years earlier than was the case a generation or two ago.

Many would agree that there is no finer feeling of special friendship than when a young man and woman agree to share their life. They then learn to live together, learn to love together, bring up children, work together against the problems of life. These are the things to aim for.

Why copy Casanova? Anyway, he got syphilis.

Emotional and Psychological Factors

By Dr. A. R. K. Mitchell,
Consultant Psychiatrist,
Fulbourn Hospital, Cambridge.

AS Dr. Statham rightly points out at the beginning of the book, we cannot fully understand sexually transmitted diseases, or any other disease for that matter, unless we consider the medical aspects involved in relationship to psychological and social factors. We must not forget that diseases happen to people and that people are not isolated from each other but interact in groups.

There is an unfortunate tendency in medicine to talk and to think as if disease processes took place in a vacuum: we talk about gonorrhoea or syphilis as if they had a separate existence; as if the pathogenic infecting agent could exist without the host. We tend to forget that the disease is neither the infecting agent nor the host, but the disease as we recognise it is the interaction between an infection agent and the host organism it infects.

People suffer from diseases and people live in groups. You are not isolated from other people—you affect them and they affect you. Whatever happens to you releases feelings; sometimes of pleasure, but often of fear. How you are feeling now influences how you relate to others around you and this ultimately influences how they come to feel about you.

We all talk and behave as if we were machines involved in events, but we are not just machines, we are people. The difference is that as far as we know, machines do not have feelings about themselves or about other machines. Certainly machines can be built which monitor their own performance, that is change their own behaviour according to what is happening around them. A thermostat is a good example: this is a machine which either operates in one direction raising the temperature, or operates in the other direction lowering the temperature, depending on information it receives about the temperature of the environment around it. A thermostat responds but it does not think or feel about what is happening in the same sense that we do. When we are in a heated argument we respond to the emotional temperature of the group, but respond as well to our own response of what is happening. What is more, most of the time we are aware that we are doing it. So human beings are different from machines in that they think and feel for themselves, and more importantly they are aware that they are doing so.

I have said that for most of the time we are aware of what we are doing and why, but what about the rest of the time? We are not always directly aware of our feelings nor of our actions and their motivation. We are influenced by unconscious factors. Not everyone is prepared to accept that these unconscious factors exist but if we look at our own experience we will find constantly recurring evidence of the operation of these unconscious factors.

Take, for example, spontaneous likes and dislikes. We say that we liked him on sight but not her, or we chose this dress rather than another. When asked why we often cannot justify our choice, all that we can say is that we just prefer this to that. Later however, we may come to realise what lay behind our choice. At the time of making it, our choice was strongly influenced by factors of which we were unaware at the time, but which can later occur to us. What was unconscious has now become conscious. Or take a further example—forgetting someone's name. It is on the tip of your tongue, you know that you know it, but you cannot recall it just at this moment. Forget all about it and sometime later the name flashes into your mind. Now you know it, you knew that you knew it so where was it when you could not recall it? It was in the unconscious or sub-conscious part of your mind. We are only beginning to realise how important these unconscious factors are in determining our conscious behaviour. Sometimes they enrich our lives; sometimes they lead to disastrous consequences.

Psychologists like Freud and Jung have shown us that the human mind is divided into three parts. First of all, the conscious part that we are well aware of, the part that carries our thoughts and feelings of the moment, and which can also recall feelings and thoughts from the past, and even project them into the future, making an estimate of how we will likely think and feel in given circumstances. Then there is the sub-conscious, or pre-conscious mind which contains thoughts and feelings not immediately accessible to consciousness, but which we can recover with a little effort.

The name you just stored away or the telephone number lies in your sub-conscious mind until you want to recall it at a particular time. By thinking carefully you can retrieve the information from your memory store. You can retrieve not only facts but feelings which belong to another place and to another time. Finally, there is the unconscious mind which is a great store-house of energy containing thoughts and feelings locked away which we cannot retrieve at will, but which in dreams and in other disguised forms slip out into consciousness in their own time, but which nevertheless continue to influence the behaviour of our sub-conscious and our conscious minds.

Freud tended to think of the unconscious as a great dark continent in which we keep imprisoned thoughts and feelings unacceptable to the conscious mind. There has therefore to be a very strong guard between the conscious and the unconscious to keep these forbidden and unacceptable elements locked into their place. It is this guard which stops us being able to reach down into the unconscious part of our experience whenever we want to. Jung on the other hand, saw the unconscious in a much more creative light, believing it to be the source of inspiration, but one which spoke in symbols. To understand our unconscious and benefit from it we have therefore to learn to tune into it and then to translate the symbolic messages which come from it into a direct and practical one.

The relevance of all this to our topic is that we cannot understand fully our sexual life and everything that goes with it, such as sexually transmitted diseases, unless we take into account these emotional factors and especially these processes which are unconscious and of which we are therefore largely unaware in our everyday lives. To develop our theme I would like to begin by looking directly at sexually transmitted diseases and the reactions which people show to them, both conscious and unconscious and then go on to look at the psychological and social aspects which lie behind the very practical questions which Dr. Statham has discussed.

V.D. Explained

Reactions to disease. We begin with two facts. Sexually transmitted disease is an infection and it is an infection contracted through sexual intercourse. Most people react to infection as something unpleasant: an infecting agent gets into the person's body and he becomes infected (unclean) as a result. The actual disease can produce skin rashes, sores or a discharge, all of which are not only unpleasant but a public declaration of being infected. Thus the person not only knows that he is unclean but feels that everyone else knows it too.

The reaction to feeling personally unclean is a reaction of *guilt*; the reaction to feeling that this is public knowledge is a reaction of *shame*. The fact that this infection is contracted through sexual contact makes the situation doubly worse, because there is still a commonly held view that sex is "not nice". Thus the reactions of guilt and shame are reinforced.

Where does this sin of "dirt" come from? Undoubtedly, some of it is an aesthetic reaction—people react against menstrual blood and genital secretions, either because of their odour or their associations of being unclean. Again, there are deeply rooted ideas that sexual contact is a very dangerous thing which has to be surrounded by taboos—these are universally accepted rules of behaviour which can only be broken at a great personal risk. A strong sense of right and wrong coupled to an awareness of one's own biological urges to break these rules means that sexual guilt is almost inevitable.

We are only too aware that strong forces inside us impel us on to do those things which we have been forbidden to do. There is also the idea that it is wrong to have biological sexual urges. Our sexual feelings as human beings have tended to be split off in our thinking into two opposite and often opposing components—love and lust. Love is seen as something pure and romantic which describes a unique relationship between two persons and is worshipped in its purest form—platonic love. At the opposite end of the spectrum we have lust which is man's animal passion which requires to be controlled and subjugated lest it destroy those involved. Love creates, lust destroys. Love and lust—agape and Eros, divine inspiration and animal appetite.

This also parallels the way we conceive of women. They are either seen as the good Earth Mother, the creator and the provider and the beginner of all things and is known in the religious setting as the Virgin Mary who bears the Holy Child without any direct sexual contamination; or else they are seen as the prostitute, the fallen woman by which man can appease his animal appetites. It is the lustful prostitute aspect of sexuality which carries the deepest sense of guilt and shame and is seen as the denial of our capacity for divine love.

In reality, both are aspects of the one whole. Sexuality is both divine and passionate. The one aspect implements the other. In our anxiety and uncertainty, we tend to divide the basic unity, split one component off from the other, and then emphasise one as a means of denying the other. We are as likely to be hurt if we see all women as angels as if we see them all as devils.

Let us now return to sexually transmitted disease and try to follow through the emotional feelings, an experience someone has who finds himself a victim of this disease. It all begins with a sexual relationship in which there is genital contact. The particular act is perhaps forgotten and then some weeks or months later symptoms and signs begin to appear and Dr. Statham has described these in detail. Gradually the suspicion that these features might mean disease begins to form in the person's mind.

The first reaction is one of denial "no, it can't be that, it couldn't happen to a person like me." It cannot be, it couldn't happen are ways of saying "I hope that it hasn't happened. I hope that it will never happen to me." But as the features progress the suspicion becomes stronger and can no longer be denied. He may even at this stage look up books in the public library or ask a friend about "a friend of his who went with this girl, etc."

These are attempts to get information without committing himself. This rarely works, so the person makes a decision to consult his doctor whom he will ask either to confirm or to refute his suspicions. There is a brief feeling of relief: there is someone to turn to for help; someone who will know what is to be done. But soon, there are feelings of vague anxiety—"how will I face him with my suspicions? What will he think of me? Will he possibly reject me as someone he doesn't want to know, someone who is unclean?"

Consulting the family doctor in these circumstances is as bad if not worse than going to the dentist, pain is anticipated, but here it is psychological pain rather than physical pain. Some can stand physical pain much more readily than psychological pain. Physical pain stops eventually; psychological pain may mean that it is difficult afterwards to go on living with yourself or with others who know your guilty secret.

All these feelings of apprehension are intensified in the consultation, but again comes the relief of certainty even if it is the certainty of confirmation of his fears, "yes, it is a disease." But with this message comes another "yes, you can be treated and cured." It is often when the patient goes home and reflects on his situation that the old fears begin to return. He goes over and over the experience as he sees it, but not necessarily as it was in reality. What he sees is *private lust* (contact with the sexual partner) followed by *public confession* (consultation with his doctor) followed by *public condemnation* (confirmation of the infection).

There then follows a succession of feelings—guilt, shame, disgust, fear and anger. He feels guilty because he believes he has broken the sexual taboo and that he is being punished as a result. All the advice given to him by parents and teachers and incorporated into his conscience nags at him. "It's all your fault. Don't tell us that we didn't warn you. You deserve all you get." He feels guilty because he knows that he is infected and feels that he is a dirty person, with a dirty body and a dirty mind. Shame follows hard on guilt. He feels *ashamed* when he knows that others see that he is guilty. The doctor knows what he has been up to, and the doctor knows what has happened as a result. What is more, he knows the doctor knows that he knows the doctor knows, and so shame and guilt pile up on top of him.

He becomes disgusted with himself and disgusted with the source of his infection, both the girl and the passion that led to him being at risk. He feels both that he is corruption (infection) and liable to corrupt (infect) others, but also that he has been corrupted by someone else. This shatters any myth that he may have of his own invincibility. He has to face up to the fact that he is just as human as the rest of us; just as liable to get into trouble and do foolish things as the next person. One of his mental defence mechanisms has been demolished. He has to face himself in all his nakedness and as a result he feels *fear*.

What other defences may now come crashing down? What other ugly truths about himself may he have to face? Has he been damaged by the infection? Will he get better? Will it be painful? Will it leave its mark on him? Will there be any long term results? Will he be sterile, will he be impotent, will he go mad, will he even die? But fear soon gives way to *anger*. He feels that he has been the object of an attack on his person and that it is not his fault, he did not ask for it. It was all that girl's fault. She is the infected one, she is the one to blame, thus once more denial is being used as a mechanism to get rid of feelings which are all too painful to bear in consciousness.

At this point some of you may well be saying to yourselves that all this is highly dramatised; that it cannot be as bad as all that. Surely people with these diseases don't go about with such feelings. In one sense if you are saying this, you will be right. Most patients are not clearly aware of their feelings, far less are they able to put them down in words.

These reactions are partly conscious, partly unconscious. How much a given patient is aware depends on how secure he is in himself and how much he can face up to, at any one time, the realities of his situation. We all carry within us a considerable capacity for infinite self-deceptions. All that many patients may feel is an unformed unrest, agitation or anxiety of which no clear expression is possible if left to themselves but given the opportunity and the encouragement to do so, the same patients will begin to talk of their guilt, their shame and their disgust. They will begin to show signs of their fear and their anger.

Those questions again. Now let us look behind those questions Dr. Statham listed early in this book to the emotional aspect which prompted them. In some of the questions this emotional aspect is fairly obvious, in others it is not so. This approach is based on the assumption that when we ask questions we are asking the questions at two levels and that we expect the answers to be at these two levels as well. The first level is a straightforward one asking for information of a factual nature—answers to the basic questions of how, why, where and how much? The second level is less declared but no less important because of that. This is the emotional level which deals with our anxieties and our fears and which seeks answers and terms of reassurance and comfort.

It is interesting that this second level may not be recognised either by the questioner or by the person who gives the answers, and yet as well as the demand for factual information, this demand for emotional reassurances may be met quite adequately without either knowing consciously this has happened. When a little boy asks a traffic warden if he can cross the road, he is not only asking about traffic density, relative velocity of the vehicles and the direction of maximum traffic flow, he is also asking if it is all right to cross at that moment. Will he be safe, will he get to the other side without coming to harm and will the kindly traffic warden act for him in a generally protective way?

Let us take Dr. Statham's questions and look specifically for the emotional undertones and the hidden anxieties.

What are sexually transmitted diseases? Again, this looks on the surface just like a specific question seeking information. But "sex" is the key emotional word. These are diseases linked in some way with sexual activity. Therefore all the anxiety and uncertainty which we have considered about sexual behaviour will be transferred on to this question. Sexual implies something at the one time mystical and magical, but at the same time earthy and private, perhaps sordid even. Thus, these diseases in their turn will have both mystical and very revolting aspects.

Can I catch them? This question really asks "Am I at risk." What are the chances that this unpleasantness, which is therefore threatening, can happen to me? Behind this lie more basic questions on the nature of disease, why some people are more prone than others, why man is diseased in the first place, questions to do with our own mortality. We do not like to think of death, neither do we like to think of illness. These are things that happen to other people—or do they? Can I really be at risk as well? The word "catch" is interesting in this context. I think it is really operative in a passive rather than an active sense. I do not want to go out and catch this in the sense of capturing something. I am really afraid that I am the one that is going to be caught, going to be captured in the grip of something which I do not really understand. The feeling is one of helplessness and vulnerability. At a sexual level, therefore, there are all the deepest fears of being harmed in some way—a woman fears being hurt by being penetrated, the man fears he may lose his manhood as the woman grasps him in the embrace of love-making.

How can I avoid them? The crucial word is "avoid". If I am at risk in this basic way, how can I protect myself? How can I recognise the people who are most dangerous to me? At a simple level, how can I recognise the "dirty people" within whom lurks this hidden danger? I do not want to be alone, but if I am to mix with others, how can I recognise who is safe and who is not? If I have strong sexual impulses inside me, how can I know if I am safe even?

Which is the serious disease? and will it make me sterile or incapable of intercourse? These questions I think are linked closely together and reflect parental injunctions with a threat of dire consequences if these injunctions are disobeyed. "Do not do that. If you do, you will go blind, you will go mad . . ." or whatever penalty seems appropriate. If you go with that kind of person you are at risk of getting an infection if you do that kind of thing together. The behaviour is forbidden and if the injunction is disobeyed, there will be serious consequences. These consequences in this setting are not too far-fetched. Sexually transmitted disease might cause genital damage and so make a person sterile or incapable of further intercourse. But the fear is exaggerated in proportion as are sanctions against certain forms of forbidden behaviour and excesses. Sexual taboos are strong laws which carry severe penalties if they are transgressed. The fear is a fear of punishment, as much as a fear of rational consequences of a particular act.

Can I be cured? This is not only a direct question regarding the nature of help available, but contains within it a request for reassurance that all will be well, not only if I get infected, but if I break the sexual taboos. I not only want to know that I can be made better by the power of medicine, but I want to know that I can be forgiven and that getting infected will not be held against me in some kind of way. I want a cure from the infection and a guarantee against social ostracisms. I want to be sure that I can be one of *us* again, having been for a time, one of *them.*

What do I look for? Prevention is better than cure. "Show me how I can be on my guard against this kind of trouble." The question implies that a kind of constant vigilance is necessary and the price to be paid to avoid the guilt which follows a social slip-up. If we are careful we need not get into that kind of difficulty, we do not have to get an infection or be hurt in some other way. We can take precautions and protect ourselves. But if we do slip up and are unlucky what are the first signs or the early signs of the infection, so that we can go quickly for treatment before matters get out of hand.

How are clinics run? The word "clinic" has a comforting medical sound about it, a place where people are helped by doctors and nurses, but it also has an impersonal sound about it—impersonal in the sense of getting on with the problem in a non-emotional and an effective way. People need both the reassurance of effective treatment, but also of a non-involving treatment. People are looking for helpers who will be sympathetic and understanding but non-judgmental. In this sense, well run clinics are both effective and protective.

What happens when I attend a clinic? This question follows on from the one before. "If I go to such a clinic, what can I expect to happen to me?" The unknown is always threatening. But also there is the question of confidence. If I trust myself to such a clinic, will I be looked after, and will my interests be looked after? Who will need to know about me and to know what I have been doing? Will I be treated with confidence and with respect?

How long do I have to attend? This asks what is involved. "What am I committing myself to if I ask for treatment." "How much will I have to give in terms of confession, trust, time, effort to get there, etc?" In a very general sense it is asking "what will I have to pay (in the way of a penalty) for getting infected if I desire to be cured and reinstated into society?"

Will my family doctor know? Will my boss/workmates get to know? and *Do letters get sent to my home?* These three questions are linked by a common theme, that of publicity. "Will what has happend to me, be made known to others?" Each of us feels guilty when we have done something which we know to be wrong. Each of us feels anxious if we feel that we are at risk. But each of us feels shame and embarrassment if both our sin and our weakness are made obvious to others. Guilt is a private emotion, whilst shame is a public emotion. We can feel shame with two levels of people. First of all with parental figures. Here the shame is of being a "bad child", of having broken the parental injunctions we have already mentioned. But with the shame comes fear of punishment. Then we feel shame with our peer group—those of our own age or circumstances. Here the shame is of "having let the side down" with fears of rejection as a consequence. You are no longer one of the boys, go away we don't want you any more. The family doctor and boss are obvious parental figures. Workmates and one's own family are peer group figures.

Can it affect my wife or girl-friend? There is not only the realistic fear of infecting other people, but once one feels a bad person there is often a concern as to whether the "badness" can escape and affect others. People often feel that psychological badness can be caught in the same way as infectious badness. If one hands on an infection or infects others with one's own badness, then there is both self-reproach and a fear of being reproached by others, of being blamed for letting one's own badness escape and hurt others. So to the fear of personal isolation is added the fear of public isolation. There is also the idea that the badness will result in splitting up two people who are important to each other—the husband/wife team, the boy-friend girl-friend alliance. The fear is of the forbidden act being punished by the severance of an important emotional bond. "Because you have been bad, you will now lose her and her love."

Are these diseases on the increase? Once more, there is not only the desire for factual information, but a desire for emotional reassurance. If these diseases are not increasing, we do not have so much to worry about. If they are increasing, what can we do to control this increase? There is a desire not only to control the spread of infection but the desire to control the impulses which lead to lack of personal control in the first place. Teach us how we can control our sexual feelings, so that we only have sexual relationships in a safe way, with no fear of infecting each other. Teach us how to control these deep-seated emotional powers that can so easily sweep us off our feet, possibly to our own destruction or the destruction of others.

Why are these diseases increasing? Under this heading Dr. Statham discusses what is popularly known as a concept of the sick society. Here, we are looking at social and emotional factors which are operating in the group rather than in the individual. There is a certain attraction in this, in that we can feel less personally involved if we are considering group behaviour rather than individual behaviour. We can if we wish dissociate ourselves from the group, while at the same time continuing to criticise it. This is another more sophisticated version of Us and Them. They are the group which do these unpleasant things. We, that is you and I and our friends, are of course quite different. Even if we do not opt out of involvement in this way, there is still a dilution of personal guilt when we consider corporate guilt.

Dr. Statham picks out a number of themes and we should look again at each in turn.

(*a*) *Prosperous insecurity:* Even though we have more material affluence, or even because of it, certain members of our society feel that they have to rebel and reject commonly accepted standards of behaviour. Affluent conformity can be very disturbing to those who require to struggle against the establishment. To be deviant is to be safe, to be conforming is tantamount to being good.

(*b*) *Increased promiscuity and experimentation:* young people want to find out for themselves, and so they reject the morality of the establishment which says "you shall do this, you shall not do that". They cling together for mutual support, doing their own thing while they find out what life is about, so that they may establish their own code of morality for themselves. It may well in the end turn out to be the same as that of the establishment, but they have come to it by themselves, not by being told what to do, or what to think.

(*c*) *Coloured immigrants:* while there may well be a realistic factor here, it may also represent the mechanism of scape-goating. That is, looking for someone else to blame for what is happening. When we scape-goat, we look for someone as different as possible from ourselves. It is not us who would do this kind of thing; it is those people over there (not at all like us) who are at fault.

(*d*) *Social isolation:* when people are lonely, they crave for intimate contact with other human beings. Barriers of language and customs can keep people apart, but the language and customs of love-making are pretty well universal with interesting local variations. This is also a game that two can play, whether it be homosexual or heterosexual. Masturbation as a social comfort has decided limitations.

(*e*) *Prostitution:* this is a form of ritualised sexual contact whereby there can be sexual release without personal commitment to the other person, other than on a financial basis. Even if prostitution is decreasing, it can still be a way in which one infected person can transmit a disease to a large number.

(*f*) *Population mobility:* people are on the move more than they used to be. Transport is easier and cheaper and more efficient. The world is truly becoming a smaller place as we can travel from one end to the other within the space of 24 hours. Air travel means that infections can be transmitted rapidly from one part of the world to another. Once the infection is noted in one passenger it is too late—he has already infected others who are well on their way to their differing destinations. Even within one country people move around as they chase after jobs or promotion prospects. We are no longer tied to mother's apron strings, nor to the maternal home as once we were. Travel may broaden the mind, but it can lead to social isolation—people are too busy going places to put down roots and to relate to each other—ships that pass in the night, casual sexual contact, spread of infection.

(*g*) *Social ignorance:* with people moving about so much, there may not be the time or the opportunity to acquaint them of the dangers of everyday life. In the rapidly developing technological society, it can so easily be taken for granted that everyone knows about contraception, sexually transmitted diseases, the dangers of drug addiction. But do they? Even if they do, there is still that pernicious emotionally determined defence—"it won't happen to me". Disaster is always what happens to other people.

(*h*) *Group pressures:* no man is an island entire unto himself—he is constantly relating to other people who are relating to him. We move through life from one group to another—the family, the neighbourhood, school, one's job, the club, one's friends. Always in each group are insidious pressures to belong, to conform to the behaviour of the group. A few wild ones rebel and escape, but most of us capitulate and give in, or perhaps only make a token bid to be that little bit different, declaring all the time that we really belong to the group. If the group we belong to believe in promiscuity, experimentation, sleeping around, then we will be promiscuous, we will experiment, we will sleep around with a very much greater risk of picking up sexually transmitted diseases.

We have now considered the emotional and psychological aspects which underline our reactions to sexual behaviour and the eventuality of becoming involved and damaged as a result.

These factors operate at a deep level in all of us because they are concerned with the very survival of our being, and with our sense of personal value and of group value. We are not aware of them in our everyday lives but they influence us all the same. When things go wrong, we can begin to catch a glimpse of them in our reactions to what has happened, but even then much remains hidden, but not without affect on us and those with whom we come in contact.

A Practical Summary

(1) Sex diseases are spread by promiscuity. They can be avoided by creating a stable relationship so that each member of a partnership is confident that the other partner is faithful. It may take many months to build up such confidence in each other.

A fully enjoyable sexual life is not achieved in " sleeping around". Given time together, a couple can instruct each other as to which techniques give most satisfaction. In this way, with their growing experience of each other, they can bring sexual fulfilment to a peak far in excess of the pleasures of earlier attempts, exciting though these may have seemed. Such a mature relationship shows casual sex to be less than second rate. (They say that stolen fruit is sweet. More often, it is not even ripe!)

(2) Loop and pill contraceptives may promote promiscuity in some women. They are no protection against sex disease. A sheath or condom is an additional precaution provided, of course, it is used throughout the sex act.

(3) Too much sexual liberty can eventually become a bore and take the enjoyment out of the process. Too much experiment and variation can have the same effect. Some people think it is a joke or clever to engage in abnormal sexual practice and relations. This is quite untrue and such misguided practice may do much to spoil your sexual life in the future.

(4) Masturbation is not abnormal. Petting is not abnormal: they can provide some sexual outlet without the risk of unwanted pregnancy and sexually transmitted disease. However both practices can be overdone and are no substitute for healthy normal sexual relationship as a part of a settled, shared life together.

(5) Sex may be a powerful force: it isn't everything, although it seems to be at times. Do not be urged or bullied into making a mess of things by pressures from others. Do not believe all you hear. Do not think that a reputation of great sexual performance when at 15 or 16 years old makes you a "big" man or a "real" woman. It often makes you merely foolish and can cause a lot of suffering.

Further Reading

Venereal Diseases, R. S. Morton (Pelican, 1966).

Postscript

THE word "chastity" has almost disappeared from the
English language, said the Rector of Treeton, Yorkshire
(the Rev. C. Dennis George), in a recent issue of his
parish magazine. He was warning young people about
sexually transmitted diseases—and many of us in the
medical profession and social services will echo his views.

"The whole concern now seems to be", the Rector's
article went on, "not whether a person remains chaste
but how we should prevent them from having babies or
abortions. There is scarcely a single word about the
shocking dangers of sexually transmitted disease, which is
usually caught through illicit intercourse.

"There is also no mention of the wreckage of human
lives, when a person finds out they have been let down by
the one to whom they gave themselves and promised so
much. All this is part of a general break-up of moral
standards."

The article continues: "It is tragic to see so many
young people marrying just because a baby is on the way.
Often they have neither money now, nor the hope of the
money adequately to support themselves. This often
means a long spell of financial hardship and a growing
bitterness and hostility, so often culminating in the break-
up of another marriage with all its misery."

Index

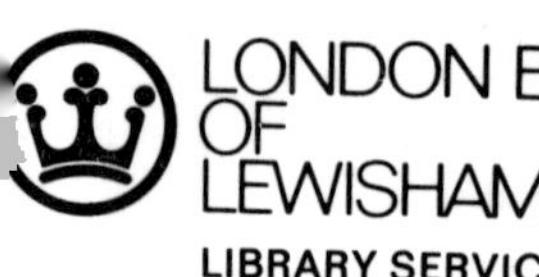

LONDON BOROUGH OF LEWISHAM

LIBRARY SERVICE

Author

Title